FUELLING BODY, MIND AND SPIRIT
A Balanced Approach to Healthy Eating

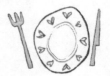

FUELLING BODY, MIND AND SPIRIT

A Balanced Approach to Healthy Eating

MIRIAM HOFFER

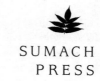

SUMACH
PRESS

NATIONAL LIBRARY OF CANADA CATALOGUING IN PUBLICATION

Hoffer, Miriam
  Fuelling body, mind and spirit: a balanced approach to healthy
eating / Miriam Hoffer.

ISBN 1-894549-27-9

1. Women—nutrition. I. Title.

TX361.W55H64 2003   613.2'082
C2003-901684-6

Edited by Sibylle Preuschat
Illustration/Cover Art © Chum McLeod/i2iart.com
Production assistance by Beverly Deutsch

Figure 6, Canada Food Guide: Source: *Canada's Food Guide
to Healthy Eating,* Health Canada, 1992 8. Reproduced with
the permission of the Minister of Public Works and
Government Services Canada, 2002.

*Sumach Press acknowledges the support of the Canada Council
for the Arts and the Ontario Arts Council for our publishing program.
We acknowledge the Government of Ontario through the Ontario
Media Development Corporation's Ontario Book Initiative.*

ONTARIO ARTS COUNCIL
CONSEIL DES ARTS DE L'ONTARIO

Printed and bound in Canada

Published by

SUMACH PRESS

1415 Bathurst Street, Suite 202
Toronto ON Canada M5R 3H8
sumachpress@on.aibn.com
www.sumachpress.com

*Dedicated to
the Wise Women at Health Watch
with whom I work.*

*I would like to thank my mother,
who started me on my path, my father, who guides
me with his vision, and my readers, John Hoffer,
Barbara Kahan and Guy Ewing.
A special thank you to Sibylle Preuschat
and to the women of Sumach Press.*

Contents

A Dietitian Challenged by Diets
Don't Be Fooled by "Diet Magic"
Diet — Belittling and Disrespectful

CHAPTER 4: *Carbohydrate, Fat, Calcium and Vitamins 67*
Carbohydrate
Fat
Calcium
Multivitamin-Mineral Supplements

CHAPTER 5: *Overcoming Barriers to Good Nutrition 74*
Lack of Time
Overcoming the Time Barrier
The Pressure To Be Thin
Resisting the Pressure To Be Thin
The Inability to Apply Knowledge to Ourselves
Overcoming the Inability to Apply Knowledge to Ourselves
Building Self-Esteem

Part 2
Fuelling the Mind and Spirit:
The Wise Women of Health Watch

INTRODUCTION 97

CHAPTER 6: *Fuelling Change:*
The Factors that Motivate Healthy Choices 100
Fear of Illness
Ageing
Weight Concerns
Children's Health
Partners
Advice From Others
Love of Life

Introduction

I am a dietitian. I work in an outpatient clinic called Health Watch, part of Women's College Hospital in Toronto, Ontario. I have been a dietitian for many years and as a result I have read, and I continue to read, about nutrition. I never had any intention of contributing another publication to the numerous nutrition books already available. The nutrition message has been explained many times over. So why, then, am I now writing yet another nutrition book after all?

The answer lies in my personal history. I started working part time at Women's College Hospital in 1990 after spending several years at home with my children. I was initially hired as a clinical dietitian to assist hospitalized people with their specialized diets. In 1994, an opening became available at Health Watch, one of the clinics at Women's College Hospital, when the dietitian who worked there took maternity leave. As I was the only dietitian in the hospital working part time, and as Health Watch operates only in the mornings, the job was offered to me. Initially I thought that in my new position at Health Watch my role would simply be to explain nutrition to the people who came to the clinic (mainly women). However, it very quickly became clear to me that in my conversations with the healthy and articulate patients of Health Watch, a dialogue usually unfolded. I talked about nutrition, and my patients told me stories about their lives. As I found myself increasingly moved and excited by what they had to say, I realized that what I was hearing were my patients' strategies for healthy living. I noticed that one woman after another had similar things to say. I felt that I was benefiting from hearing my patients' views. It struck me that others might benefit as well.

With the hospital's permission, I began taking a tape recorder to work and recording my conversations with those women who consented to share their thoughts on tape. At home, I tried to organize what I was being told in a way that made sense to me. I wanted to put down on paper all the knowledge and wisdom about how to stay healthy expressed by my patients, organize it into readable form, and offer the result back to the clinic. I often tell my patients that I am a link between them and the next patient, that is, I take the advice each person gives me and I offer it to the next. My initial impetus for writing this book was to create a more expanded and formalized version of that daily process.

But the dietitian in me was also listening. I noticed how common certain eating patterns were in the women I was counselling, and how that pattern was reinforced by worries about body weight. I also noticed that although many of my patients were knowledgeable about nutrition, something was preventing them from eating the way they knew was healthy. What were the barriers keeping my patients from achieving healthy eating habits? How could I explain nutrition in such a way as to overcome those barriers? How could I organize my thoughts so that they would make sense to most people?

I have combined these two purposes into this book. I will present the wisdom of the women of Health Watch that has so impressed me. And I will explain, just as I do to my patients, how to sustain health with good eating habits — habits that respect the fact that food supplies not only vitamins, minerals and fibre, but energy, our fuel for living. I hope that the final result you hold in your hands will provide you with "fuel" for body, mind and spirit.

I'd like to tell you now about Women's College, the hospital where Health Watch is located, because I think this has had an impact on the type of clinic we have become. Although the hospital is now called Women's College Ambulatory Care Centre and is part of Sunnybrook and Women's Health Sciences Centre, the original name still holds a special place in the hearts of the hospital's patients and staff. Women's College has played a unique role in the field of medicine in the province of Ontario. Since its earliest days at the turn of the century when it provided a haven for women doctors, Women's College has been a leader in Ontario's health care community. Today it provides service to men and women, and is staffed by men as well as women. It continues to provide leadership in developing and supporting education programs, research studies and care protocols specific to women. It also has been supportive of its staff and of individual initiatives they might undertake, perhaps because for most of its history it has been a small hospital. It is a hospital that has traditionally given personal attention to patients in a warm and caring environment. The name Women's College Hospital evokes emotional reactions in people who received care there. After I gave a talk one day at a seniors' residence, a woman came up to me, touched my sleeve, and said, "My husband died at Women's College Hospital." She clearly wanted to feel a connection to the hospital through me.

Health Watch started life over fifty years ago as the Cancer Detection Centre. It was one of only two sites in Ontario where pap smears were done, and women flocked from all over the province to receive this "personal" test from a female-centred, female-staffed clinic. In 1993, through the vision of the nurse manager of the clinic and with the support of the hospital, Health Watch adopted its current name, and its focus also shifted.

Today the clinic is much more than a cancer detection centre. It can best be described as a wellness centre that serves both men and women, although it is still mainly women who come. Much of the appeal for the women patients lies in the fact that the clinic is staffed by women physicians. On their annual visit, patients receive a complete physical exam that can include a pap test, a breast exam and an examination of moles. The doctor addresses particular medical concerns patients may have and discusses menopausal, sexual or emotional issues. Blood work may be ordered if deemed necessary, to check hemoglobin levels, for example. Mammograms are ordered according to current guidelines. Bone density scans are also ordered if needed. Referrals to specialists can be made. We show health-related videos, on topics such as breast self-examination and dealing with urinary incontinence. A dietitian (myself), a nurse, and a physiotherapist are on staff and offer specialized information. Health Watch is a place where people can get a complete physical exam and extensive health-related information in a safe, supportive environment, knowing that all aspects of their health will be explored and discussed.

Dr. Rohan Maharaj spent six months in our clinic as a Women's Health Scholar while working on his Master of Health Science degree at the University of Toronto in 1998. In a paper based on unpublished research conducted at Health Watch, *Why Do Women Seek Preventive Care from a Specialized Clinic?*, he concludes:

> All of the interviewees had experienced a negative personal experience with their own Family Physician or through family or friends with the traditional health system. The women felt they would get a thorough exam at the clinic and all aspects of women's health would be addressed. The name Women's College Hospital was very important even if they saw a male physician. Getting a full report of their results for their own records, the educational features such as breast self exam techniques and the dietitian consultation, were all positive factors in their decision to continue attending the clinic.

As Dr. Maharaj's findings indicate, the people who come to Health Watch are a select population. They have indicated by their presence at the clinic that they are interested in their health. They range in age from nineteen to ninety-one, with the majority being in the menopausal years of forty-five to sixty-five. Many of the people who come have read extensively on the subject of health, are already exercising and eating well and are often taking vitamin and mineral supplements. Although they have had their share of diseases, including cancer, heart disease and depression, the women who come are, for the most part, healthy. They value the role Health Watch plays in helping them stay well. As Helen, 42, says, "Coming to Health Watch creates a mental commitment to listen." Heather, 56, who gets a lower life insurance rate because she comes in every year, adds, "Health Watch is my preventive medicine." Marnie, 47, explains, "Coming to Health Watch helps you focus: you make the time to come, you fill in the form, and you know what you're supposed to do." (Note that here, and throughout the book, all of my patients' names — with the exception of one woman who did not want to be anonymous — have been changed to protect their privacy.)

Many of the women I see at the clinic are from rural areas where access to health care is not easy to obtain. The majority travel two hours or more to get here. Many are on a waiting list for a family doctor in their area. Those who do have a doctor may come to the clinic if they don't feel entirely comfortable with that individual. As one woman said to me, "My physician is my next door neighbour." Given that situation, she definitely did not want him to do her pap tests. Many of our patients also use the clinic to tap into Toronto's community of specialists. The clinic's patients drive through winter snows and summer heat. They rise early in the morning to make their appointments on time, they take a day off work, and they find substitute caregivers for family members. They bring their family, their friends, and their workmates, and they've started to bring their husbands and their sons — but women still make up 98 percent of our patient base.

When the clinic shifted its focus from cancer detection to wellness, a dietitian was hired to promote the role of nutrition in health maintenance and disease prevention. I started filling this role in 1994.

Working at Health Watch has presented me with a professional challenge. I'd like to explain this with reference to my personal career history. I've always had an interest in nutrition. In fact, I became acquainted with the principles of good nutrition at an early age and this I attribute to my mother. Although we had the usual "treats" in the house and my mother was very fond of chocolate, she never served a meal that didn't include a vegetable. For those of us who did not care for cooked vegetables, she always had some raw ones available. A special treat that she often brought home from the grocery store for me were peas in the pod. My mother maintained the vegetable habit all her life. A childhood friend of mine who returned home to see her family one holiday described to me the visit she had with my parents on that trip. My mother led her into the living room, went into the kitchen, and brought out a huge raw carrot for her. My friend had to carry on a conversation with my parents while chewing on this carrot as politely and quietly as she could manage!

But despite my enthusiasm for healthy food, when I first started university I studied sociology. Somewhere along the line, however, I heard sociology defined as "the elaboration of the obvious." I was uncertain about a career in sociology. Remembering my interest in nutrition, I went back to university to study it. Well, don't I now find myself in a similar situation? Is not nutrition "obvious" to most people? Is not nutrition a subject in which we are all experts because we all eat?

This became my dilemma when I started to work at Health Watch. Not only does each person who comes to the clinic have an opinion as to what constitutes a healthy diet, she is also carrying her sister's, her friend's and her doctor's opinions as well, not to mention the often conflicting "facts" regularly presented in the popular press. So what is a healthy diet? And is there a right answer to that question?

In 1994 I thought there might be. As did the dietitian before me, I started off at Health Watch armed with my Canada's Food Guide to Healthy Eating and my Fat Scoreboard, a chart listing the fat content of various foods. My mandate, I believed, was to teach the basics of nutrition. Fat phobia was at its peak at the time, and I was right on board with monitoring my patients' fat intake. I don't remember when I stopped the routine use of the Fat Scoreboard but as I learned more about my patients' eating patterns I realized that nutrition was about more than just fat. And it didn't take long for me to realize that almost everyone already "knew" nutrition. What did I have to say about eating vegetables to an 85-year-old woman who had raised six children? What was my role? I've learned since that my role is to remind women of what they already know about nutrition and to explore the barriers that prevent them from carrying out in practice what they know in theory. And ultimately my role is to give my patients permission to relinquish the idea of a perfect diet.

I continue to listen and to learn. I also continue to be confused and beguiled by the conflicting attitudes and actions that we human beings display — and I grow ever more proud and confident in women's basic wisdom, in their ability to figure out what is right for them. It is these women of Health Watch who have taught me what you find in this book. Therefore it is to the wise women of Health Watch that I dedicate this book.

Fuelling Body, Mind and Spirit: A Balanced Approach to Healthy Eating begins with a discussion of "triangle eating," my term for the eating pattern that I've seen so many women adopt, a pattern that provides both inadequate fuel for the day's activities and often inadequate nutritional intake as well. I discuss what my patients tell me about the barriers to maintaining healthier "fuelling" patterns, and suggest ways to overcome these.

I then turn to the women of Health Watch for "mind and spirit" fuel, exploring the many wise words they have given me about how to live a fulfilled and healthy life.

An Important Note: Guilt About Eating

As my reader, you are about to encounter several chapters that detail my thoughts on how and what to eat. Before you read this material, I would like you to have an understanding of the spirit in which I wrote it.

Eating habits are personal and one of my challenges as a dietitian is approaching this private area with sensitivity. Many of my patients are defensive about their eating habits, more are apologetic. Some use references to their eating patterns to belittle themselves. I often joke with my patients that when they were born their parents were given, along with the new bundle of joy, a box to be opened as soon as the new baby was ready to receive its contents — a box of guilt! The women I see at Health Watch are already working hard, raising families, helping out parents and neighbours. The last thing they need is to burden themselves with guilt and self-blame about their eating habits. I want them to eat as well as they can, and I want to make achieving that goal as easy as possible. To that end, I want my patients and my readers to realize that there is no ideal way of eating. Simple is good. Balance is important.

In my practice I try to take away blame. Women are already saddled with too much blame — I don't want to add to the burden. I do this by pointing out the obvious to my patients: there is not enough time in a day to do every health action we are told to do; there is no such thing as a perfect diet; no one has a licence on laziness; they are not the only ones binge eating in the evenings. I do not allow self-deprecating comments. At times I will turn my pencil to the eraser end and symbolically erase, by using a rubbing motion in the air, negative thoughts that my patients express about themselves.

I am also very careful with the words I use. I try very hard not to affix blame nor to equate eating behaviour with worth. I try not to use the word "should" in my office. People can only do the best they can given any particular set of circumstances. I remind my patients that it is ironic but true that in times of extreme stress, when healthy activity and eating habits can help sustain us, few of us are able to eat well or exercise, precisely because of the stressors we are dealing with. I'll also often ask my patients if they choose their friends based on weight or eating habits. Of course they don't! I then ask them to extend the same generosity to themselves, to not reject themselves for their eating patterns or body size. As you read this book I hope you will do the same. If the advice given here makes sense to you, you will find it much easier to put it into practice if you approach change in a spirit of self-acceptance rather than self-reproach.

PART 1

FUELLING THE BODY

I

Two Ways of Eating:
Triangle Eating vs. Rectangle Eating

Women who come to Health Watch are asked to fill out a short health questionnaire. The nutrition section asks a series of questions, including the following: How many meals a day do you eat? How many cups of coffee do you drink? What is a typical day's eating pattern for you?

After many months of reading and thinking over the answers, I decided that we seem to have lost track of the primary reason we eat. We have forgotten that the main function of food is to provide fuel. Food provides us with the energy we need to get through a day as well as to do all the cellular growth and repair kinds of things that go on in the body. Hunger is our signal that we have run out of fuel. But I noticed that many of my patients had also lost the ability to recognize and respond to their bodies' hunger signals.

Of course we also benefit from the nourishment that food delivers to our bodies; we need the vitamins, minerals and other nutrients it contains to function properly. It is this second aspect of food that most health professionals focus on and that is written about repeatedly in nutrition books. And indeed, food as nourishment is truly important. But I found that my patients already knew all about this function of food. It has not become my focus at Health Watch.

Triangle Eating

What I see in my patients over and over again is a pattern of eating that delivers fuel in an unbalanced way — many of us, I believe, have what I call a fuel distribution problem. We tend to ignore our need for fuel, carry on in our day as best we can and wonder why we may feel our energy drop or why we have a ravenous appetite late in the day. To be more specific, my patients regularly admit to eating little or nothing at breakfast, ignoring lunch, and then bingeing in the evening. In fact, I have now seen this pattern of eating so frequently that I term it "triangle eating" and I often draw small triangles for people to explain how I see the way they eat. Let me try to show you how I explain triangle eating to my patients. Here's the picture as seen in Figure 1.

The area within the triangle represents the total amount of food required to meet the day's fuel requirements. The triangular shape represents the distribution of food throughout the day. The triangle's width increases as one moves toward its base, as does the amount of food eaten as the day goes on. I call the right line of the triangle, the one being navigated by the skier, the hunger line. Even if you start off the day with no food at all, you may not feel your hunger, depending on how busy you are. As the triangle's narrow

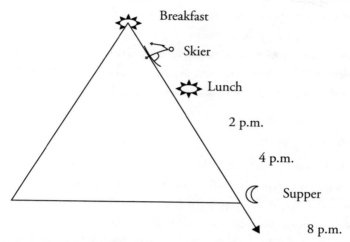

Figure 1: **Triangle Eating**

width at the top shows, you eat little or nothing. But as the day progresses, your hunger intensifies, until you can ignore it no longer. I sometimes also call this line the slippery slope of hunger, because I see that as hunger, represented by the skier, approaches the bottom of the hill, it travels faster and faster, becoming ever more difficult to ignore. In some cases the skier slips off the triangle altogether: hunger has become so "accelerated" that it causes evening eating. Of course, it is not unusual to have a larger supper meal than the other meals, but I believe that it is the size of the first meal that determines the ultimate size of the last meal. As the triangle shape demonstrates, the smaller the breakfast, the larger the supper — or the evening binge.

To make this same point, I sometimes ask my patients to imagine a person crawling across a desert without any water. When the person is finally allowed a glass of water, does she take a sip and say thank you, that was tasty? Or does she gulp down not only that glass but several more? I believe that people are crawling through a symbolic desert when they follow the triangle eating pattern. By the time they allow themselves to eat, they want large amounts of food or heavily concentrated food, and so the binge begins.

Sumo Wrestlers — Champion Triangle Eaters

There are three key daily stress points that women who are triangle eaters repeatedly identify in discussion with me. These are noted on the triangle diagram. The first one occurs around two in the afternoon, after lunch. People tell me how tired they suddenly become. Some say it is because they have eaten bread at lunch. (The anti-carbohydrate movement has a tight hold on people's minds.) Perhaps. I ask these women, "Could it be possible skipping breakfast and not eating anything until lunch causes you to run out of fuel by two o'clock?" It seems to be a very hard thing for many of my patients to accept — this idea that little or no breakfast preceding a very small lunch may not provide enough fuel. They also don't understand why, if they hardly eat any food during the day, they don't lose weight. (I'll discuss this concern later on, as well as my eventual realization that these worries about weight help drive triangle eating.)

A second key stress point arrives at four in the afternoon, when hunger hits my patients over the head. Women use the word ravenous to describe this hunger; many say they feel sugar cravings at this point in the day. Again, my patients seem to have difficulty understanding why they feel this way, or they blame themselves for a lack of control. And again, I do my best to explain that they are suffering from a fuel shortage.

Food's fuel value is measured in calories. The average woman's daily fuel requirement is between 1,800 and 2,000 calories. Many women work out three to five times a week — their fuel requirement is even higher. If we were to fuel our bodies in as consistent a pattern as we fuel our cars (not an exact analogy, I admit), we would take in a minimum of 500 to 600 calories per meal for the first two meals, amounts which allow for a slightly larger supper. For a breakfast meal that would mean eating a bowl of cereal, a cup of milk, a piece of toast with peanut butter, and some fruit. If we do not fuel our bodies in an even manner, that is, if we do not eat a sufficient breakfast and lunch, and snacks as required, then we start to feel overwhelming hunger around four in the afternoon — hunger that will continue for the rest of the day. Most people cannot resist eating once this late-day hunger hits, and they frequently binge, trying to take in enough fuel to meet their daily requirement all at one go.

Repeated regularly, such an eating pattern does not support weight loss and, in fact, might even promote weight gain, since we burn or metabolize our fuel best during the day. As day moves into night, the body slows down its metabolism and goes into calorie storage mode. Some researchers assert that metabolism also slows down when no food is consumed for several hours. I suspect that people who practise triangle eating for very many years — and I do not think this happens in the short run — start to look like triangles. Apparently this is the technique used by sumo wrestlers to achieve their large weight goals. They delay

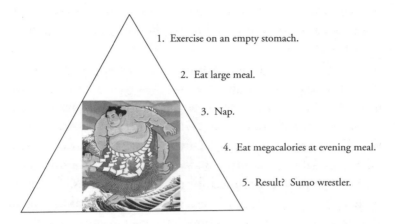

1. Exercise on an empty stomach.

2. Eat large meal.

3. Nap.

4. Eat megacalories at evening meal.

5. Result? Sumo wrestler.

Figure 2: **The Dangers of Triangle Eating**

eating until late in the morning, having exercised on an empty stomach, have a nap, and eat only one more very large meal late in the day. I've never met a woman who wants to look like a sumo wrestler. How strange then, that so many of us mimic the way these wrestlers eat! Figure 2 sums up this point about the dangers of triangle eating; it shows that consuming large amounts of food late in the day leaves us with excess, unexpended fuel.

What Are We Eating at Day's End?

Another thing I have noticed is that the food a person reaches for at four o'clock and again at eight o'clock (the third key stress point in a triangle eater's day) tends to be rich in fat. I believe that a person becomes so hungry that the only foods that can fill them quickly and with satisfaction are those rich in fat. Who hasn't searched the cupboard and fridge at night looking for that "it" we need to satisfy our hunger? Can you relate to the "No, that's not it!" scenario? Indeed, fat supplies twice the calories of carbohydrate and protein, and I believe it is natural to crave it when we are *that* hungry. When we've gone too long without fuel, we simply don't have time to waste on calorie-poor foods like vegetables, even when we realize that they may deliver more nutrients than the particular food we crave.

Many of my patients insist that they are not *that* hungry, they merely have a "sweet tooth." I tell them that I am looking at the situation through a different window, and from my vantage point I don't see what they believe to be the obvious. I look at the total picture, I explain, at the whole day, and I point out that it is not usually sugar they are craving so much as the fat. I say they have a "fat tooth."

I point out that the foods they are eating in the afternoon and evening are essentially based on fat. I explain that I classify these foods as sweet or salty "fat snacks." Sweet fat includes chocolate, cookies and pastries. People who describe themselves as having a sweet tooth eat these. People who prefer their fatty foods salty reach for cheese, chips and peanuts. I do not believe that people have an overdeveloped "sweet tooth" or that they crave salt. I believe they have a "fat tooth," created by hunger, and that they prefer their fat to be sweet or salty.

I would add here that I have talked to people who crave neither sweet nor salty foods. They, instead, tend to be meat eaters. So I have added a third category of fatty foods to my list — foods that are just plain fat. People who crave their fat unadorned eat very large portions of meat at supper, put extra salad dressing on salads and have gobs of butter on bread or potatoes.

The following table summarizes the fatty "it" foods we reach for to refuel at the end of a triangle eating day. At the far right is a brief list of meal foods we typically miss eating when we skip meals during the day and binge at night.

Table 1: "It" Foods vs. Meal Foods

Sweet Fat	Salty Fat	Plain Fat	Meal Foods
chocolate	chips	large portions	meat, poultry,
cookies	regular popcorn	of: meat gravy	fish
pastries	salty peanuts	butter, etc.	tofu
pie	cheese		beans
ice cream	nachos		vegetables/fruit
			cereal/bread

My patients insist that they eat at night because they are bored, are winding down from a busy day, have no will power. I call all cravings hunger, until proven otherwise. Of course there can be an emotional component to binge eating and this may have to be dealt with. But I ask women to first nourish themselves properly during the day — I feel this is required if they are to successfully deal with any other eating problems that might exist.

More Fibre, Less Fat

There is another reason we reach for fatty foods after a day of not eating. We tend to eat our meal foods, that is, whole grains, vegetables, and protein, at breakfast and lunch. But if you are having a small breakfast or lunch, you are limiting your meal foods. That, in turn, means you are limiting your fibre intake, because fibre is most often found in the meal foods. Fibre plays an important role in filling us — when we don't eat enough of it at meals, consumption of non-meal snack foods increases.

The point I am making here about the inverse relationship between fibre and fat intake is illustrated in the following diagram:

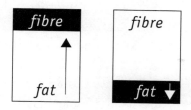

Figure 3: **Fat and Fibre in the Diet**

To repeat, as fibre intake decreases, fat intake increases. As I was working on this book my son came home from university for the weekend. More accurately, my son came home hungry. As we talked, I helped him make a snack that would tide him over until supper. As he picked some lettuce out of the salad bowl for his sandwich, I suggested he have a serving of salad as well. I think what he said next epitomizes what I am saying here about fat and fibre. Taking a small serving of salad, he explained, "I can't take any more because I don't want to spoil my appetite for non-salad." Of course, if you want to "spoil your appetite" for fatty, low-nutrient snack foods, you'll want to eat that salad and many other healthy, fibre-rich foods during the day.

Fooling Ourselves

The triangle eating I've described here is generally related to worries about weight. We fool ourselves into thinking that by eating less during the day we will achieve weight loss, even though this approach leads to evening binges. In my practice, the clearest example of how this works was provided by a patient who had cut bread out of her lunch. "I'm trying to lose weight," she said. "Oh, but I notice that you're eating ice cream and cookies in the evening!" I exclaimed.

Our self-deception is reinforced by doctors and the press. We are told over and over that in order to lose weight we have to eat less. If you're eating two pieces of toast at breakfast, say the weight loss pundits, cut back to one. During the Christmas season, we are told that if we know we're going to a buffet at night, we should eat lightly during the day. Heaven help us! I tell people that if they know they're going to a buffet at night and they don't want to overeat, they should stuff themselves silly throughout the day with healthy high fibre vegetables and fruits. By the time they get to their party, I explain, they'll be able to choose what they eat, rather than be driven to eat everything in sight because they have just crossed the desert. I also tell people that in order to weigh less, they have to eat more! Of course, I don't mean we need to consume more calories in total; I mean we need to eat sufficient amounts of meal foods during the day to satisfy our hunger and meet our fuel requirements. And our fuel requirements must be met. Just because we eat a small breakfast or lunch does not mean we don't eat. We just eat later. I tell people that a calorie not eaten before four in the afternoon is eaten after. I also tell them that a calorie eaten before four in the afternoon is burned, a calorie eaten after that time stored. I can't point to a scientific study, but remember those sumo wrestlers.

I will discuss how to go about balancing our fuel intake in detail next, when I discuss rectangle eating. I'd like to finish up my look at triangle eating with a perfect description of the pattern from one of my patients. If anything in Karen's story sounds familiar, I hope you will read on to discover how you can break the triangle eating pattern and begin enjoying the benefits of being well fed — and fuelled — all day long.

> I recognize that I need to eat regularly and I always have good intentions but I don't always do that. It depends on how my day goes. Some days I don't get away from my desk. I work at my desk so I don't eat and I come home and depending on what I've got going, I might not. When I come home at ten o'clock at night, I shovel whatever I can find in my face, box of cookies, a cake, whatever I can get. You can't go all day and not eat. On the other side, if I get up and have my yogurt with some granola in it and take my little apple to work for a break and come home at lunch and have a nice little salad, and take some veggies for the afternoon, then I can come home and eat a decent meal and go to bed. But if I don't do that, I binge.

> You've got to fill your body with those calories one way or the other and you can do it either reasonably or you fill it all in at 2,000 kilocalories all in one shot.
>
> KAREN, 45

Rectangle Eating

As we've seen, triangle eating tends to lower nutrient intake and may also contribute to the very weight gain its practitioners are trying to avoid. I believe that one of the reasons people feel so good and do not feel hungry on "fad" diets during the first few days is, in fact, because they are eating more food at breakfast and lunch. It is obvious to me that the way to overcome triangle eating is to eat more during the day. Because I encourage my patients to fill their plates at breakfast and lunch, I often refer to myself as the "eat more" dietitian. I call the eating pattern I try to encourage "rectangle eating." Rectangle eating delivers fuel at regular intervals during the day, so when we practise it, we lose our cravings, bingeing comes to an end, and our nutrient intake and overall health improve. The following diagram illustrates how rectangle eating works. Please note that the area within the rectangle is equivalent to the area within the triangle. That is, they both represent total fuel intake during the day.

I change my image here from a skier accelerating on a triangle's downward slope to a mountain climber descending a peak, represented by the rectangle. Mountain climbers get to the bottom of a mountain in a more even-paced way than skiers — they rappel down, section by section. Just as the

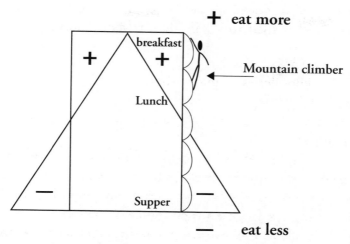

Figure 4: **Rectangle Eating**

climber descends section by section, so the rectangle eater fuels each segment of the day with healthy food, especially high-fibre plant foods. When you're a rectangle eater, you start the day with breakfast. When you're full, you stop eating. What contributes to your feeling of fullness is both the energy and fibre content of the food — the fibre, in fact, acts to physically limit the amount of food you can or want to eat at one time. When you get hungry again you eat, and so on until you reach the bottom of your rectangle where you stop your eating for the day. The diagram shows that the rectangle eater consumes more food at the day's beginning, when triangle eaters are still starving themselves. But by the day's end, when the triangle eater has generally lost control of her eating, the rectangle eater is able to stick to reasonable portions of healthy food. My patients who try rectangle eating report that their cravings and fat binges decrease.

They're also pleased by the disappearance of the afternoon fatigue that used to set in after a whole morning of fuel deprivation.

Eating Enough

When we practise rectangle eating, we finally begin eating enough.

Given the obsession many women have with losing weight, one of the hardest jobs I have, I think, is to convince my patients that they are not eating enough during the day. Some women laugh outright. Some are relieved. Some are politely silent. One woman who complained of afternoon sugar cravings came back the following year with a food diary that included much more food at breakfast and lunch. I launched into my "Isn't that wonderful!" gush. She stopped me with the words, "I didn't lose any weight." Now this didn't bother me very much because I do make an effort to tell people that I don't promise weight loss. But then she went on to say that she had lost her cravings. I was delighted. "In fact," she said, "I thought there was something wrong with you when you told me to eat more food." She hadn't believed that fuelling herself better early in the day would affect her cravings.

I have heard people coming out of my office shouting to their friends in the waiting room, "She said I don't eat enough!" I have had people thank me for telling them they can eat more. You know by now that, in fact, I'm talking about redistributing the day's fuel so that more is eaten during the day, at breakfast and lunch, so that one is able, in fact, to eat less after four in the afternoon.

Metaphors about triangle and rectangle eating aside, what I spend most of my time at Health Watch doing, really, is talking about eating normally, meaning that we eat when we are hungry and stop when we are full. I believe, as I will discuss later, that many things conspire against our ability to do this. I believe that when we eat normally, we naturally consume enough food to provide sufficient fuel throughout the day. Unlike triangle eating, normal eating does not lead to evening binges that encourage weight gain. I believe that by combining normal, healthy eating with healthy active living, both health and weight can be maintained. This idea will be discussed in more detail in the next chapter. But after months or years of triangle eating, normal, or rectangle eating, has to be relearned.

Normal eating is balanced eating: it provides both a balanced fuel intake and balanced food choices. As I've shown in my discussion of rectangle eating, not only is it important to get enough total fuel every day, but also to make sure that one's fuel intake is distributed in such a way that a steady and even supply of energy is available throughout the day. To make rectangle eating more tangible, I ask my patients to imagine taking all the food they need to eat in a day, throwing it into a bag, shaking it all up, and pulling a third of it out at a time. That is, I ask people to aim to eat a third of all the food they need for the whole day during the first third of the day (breakfast and mid-morning snack), a second third during the second part of the day (lunch and mid-afternoon snack), and the last third at supper. Each one-third portion of food needs to consist of a balanced meal.

We will see how to put together such balanced meals in the next chapter.

2

Circle Eating:
The Plate Method

We come now to our final "nutrition geometry" lesson. We will be successful at rectangle eating if we stick to the "plate method" or what might whimsically be called "circle eating." The plate method helps my patients visualize a balanced meal. To communicate what I mean by the word "meal" to my patients, I often start by asking people to think about what they would serve company for a meal. The generally accepted company meal typically includes meat (protein), potato (starch) and vegetables. (I refer to this as a balanced meal; one of my patients called it a "square" meal.) People are not likely to serve a meal to guests that is missing one of these components; even if they did, they would be aware of the fact that it was missing. Although Canada's Food Guide to Healthy Eating combines vegetables and fruit into one group of foods, I consider them two groups because of their nutritional importance, and I ask my patients to imagine adding a serving of fruit to the plate, although it is not traditionally thought of as part of a company meal, except perhaps, at dessert. The basic plate or circle of food has now been constructed in my patient's imagination. This has been illustrated by the Canadian Diabetes Association as follows:

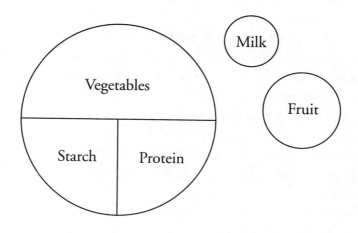

Figure 5: **A Balanced Meal**

After we've established what belongs on a plate, I ask people to use this plate method, or circle eating, to plan all three of the day's meals. At each meal, in other words, they should see protein, starch, vegetables and fruit on their plate.

Many people, of course, eat "mixed up meals." The plate method can still be used to identify the essential components of the meal even if they're not separately displayed on the plate. For example, many of the women I talk to have soup for lunch. I always ask, "What kind of soup — is it home made, is it canned, or is it a powder to which hot water is added?" I then ask them to visually pour off all the water from the soup and place what is left on a plate. I then ask them, "Is this a meal?" Vegetable soup will supply vegetables but may lack protein or starch. Canned chicken noodle soup doesn't supply enough protein, starch or vegetables. Some powdered soup broths provide little more than tasty hot water.

The protein at each meal can be animal or vegetable (examples of protein foods will follow). The starch can be a grain, that is rice, pasta, bread, or cereal, or it can be a potato. (Potatoes are, in fact, vegetables and are represented as vegetables in Canada's Food Guide. In our diets, however, they usually serve the role of starch. Food guides from Great Britain, Korea, Portugal and Germany put potatoes in the grains group rather than the vegetables group to avoid the confusion.) In any case, people who have potatoes at a meal can count the potato as both a starch and a vegetable. Vegetables and fruit can be raw or cooked, canned or frozen. The different foods that make up a balanced plate can be served together or separated. For example, many people will have fruit as a between-meal snack. To people who are not fond of fruit, I say eat extra vegetables. With people who do not like vegetables I try to find at least two or three they are willing to eat, or a preparation method that makes vegetables more palatable. Given their nutritional value, I cannot compromise on vegetables — I do believe that there are things in life one does because one is a grown-up and eating vegetables even if one dislikes them is one of those things.

I tell my patients that they don't have to eat all of their meal at one time, but that I would like them to finish that one meal before moving on to the next. Eat what you can at the meal, I explain, and what you can't finish, eat later as a snack. I encourage people who are unable to have snacks during the day due to time restrictions to eat a little more at meal times.

As you can see, circle eating is quite structured. I explain that a company meal is very structured as well. However, there is a tremendous variety of foods to choose from and the meal doesn't have to be eaten all at the same time. I like my patients to think of all of their meals as company meals — I ask them to invite themselves as a guest to each meal. I want them to value and treat themselves as they would a guest at their table.

I fine tune circle eating as follows. If the starch at a given meal is a grain food (as opposed to a potato), then I ask my patients to have two servings, not merely one. And although vegetables are part of a balanced meal, I don't ask people to have vegetables at breakfast. I do, of course, recommend fruit at breakfast or as a mid-morning snack. "But," I say, "make sure to have them at lunch. Make lunch a vegetable opportunity." One woman told me that somewhere in her mother's book of rules it said that supper had to include a vegetable and that even though her husband didn't like vegetables, she served them at that meal. I told her to add another rule about vegetables at lunch and this she under-stood. I also like to point out to people that vegetables, and grains too, for that matter, can be considered gifts of the earth and appreciated as such.

Finally, each meal should include a calcium source and some fat. (I'll discuss both calcium and fat in more detail later.)

Circle Eating in Practical Terms

So what does circle eating look like in real life?

A **breakfast** would include the following foods:

Starch: About 1 cup/250 mL whole grain cereal plus one
slice of whole wheat toast (two servings).
Protein: 1 cup/250 mL milk in the cereal (one serving).
Calcium: Supplied by the milk.
Fruit: Banana (one serving).
Fat: 1–2 tbsp/15–30 mL peanut butter on toast (optional).

No vegetables are required at breakfast. I ask women who
can't eat this much to eat what they can and have the rest as
a snack.

Lunch might look like this:

Starch: Two slices whole grain bread (equals two
servings).
Protein: 2 oz/60 g meat, fish or cheese (one serving).
Vegetables: Lettuce and tomato in the sandwich plus baby
carrots (one to two servings).
Fruit: Apple (one serving).
Calcium: The cheese in the sandwich, a small tub of
yogurt or 1 cup/250 mL of low-fat milk.

Again, I ask women who can't eat this much to eat what they
can and have the rest as a snack.

Supper might look like this:

Starch: 1 cup/250 mL rice or pasta, or one potato
(two servings).
Protein: 2–3 oz/60–90 g meat, chicken or fish, or
1/2 cup/125 mL legumes (one serving).

Vegetables: 1/2 cup /125 mL cooked broccoli plus
      1 cup /250 mL salad (two servings).
Fruit: 1/2 cup/125 mL fruit salad.
Calcium: 1 cup/250 mL low-fat milk.
Fat: 1 tbsp/15 mL salad dressing.

Please note that for most people the meals I've described here provide roughly 600 calories per meal, a minimum quantity of food. Active people will need more food than is represented by the examples given. That is, they will need three such meals daily plus one to two snacks, or they may want more servings of various foods at each meal. Snack foods can simply be more meal foods, or they can be traditional snack items. Examples of snack foods include fruit, crackers, vegetables and dip, popcorn, nuts, trail mix and cookies. I have no objection to people eating sweet treats as snacks. These foods taste good and give pleasure. I do object to people eating their snacks before they've finished their meal. The most common pattern I see is a person eating half of a sandwich for lunch in an attempt to cut calories, and then getting so hungry in the afternoon that she snacks on cookies. I tell her, "There is nothing wrong with cookies. Just finish your meal first!" My patients usually smile when I say this to them — they recognize it as advice they give to their children.

If people feel they have overeaten during the day, then they can reduce their evening intake. I tell people that if they must diet, please diet at supper, not at breakfast or lunch. It is also possible to plan meals so that only low calorie versions of most foods appear on the plate.

The approach to meal planning I present here is based on Canada's Food Guide to Healthy Eating (CFG). The Food Guide shows the food needed for a whole day; following it supplies about 1,800 calories daily. So when I ask my patients to eat a third of the day's fuel requirements at each meal, I am really asking them to eat a third of the Food Guide. The back page of the Food Guide, the one I use to illustrate my plate method, is reproduced here. It states very clearly what a serving size is.

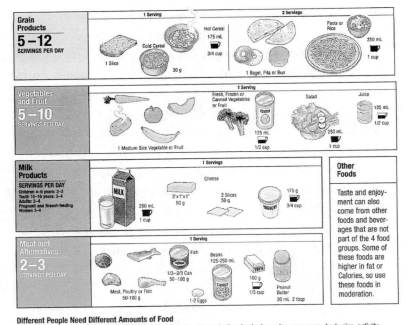

Figure 6: **Canada's Food Guide**

The Fear of Eating Too Much

When I present the plate method, or circle eating, to my patients, I find they are often afraid to eat what they consider to be so much food. Underneath that fear, of course, is the fear of weight gain. At this point I return to my explanation of triangle eating, pointing out the catch-up eating that most people do at the end of the day to make up for the food not eaten during the day. I also explain that people can play catch-up at times other than the end of the day. For very restrained eaters, catch-up can come at a time of lowered defences — perhaps on a weekend, or just before a menstrual period, when some women experience intense food cravings. The need to catch up might also contribute to stress eating. I believe — and for this I have no proof other than my clinical observations — that some women may not play catch-up until they're pregnant or menopausal. I believe that the body has a very long memory for food deprivation.

Another thing that helps my patients overcome their fear of circle eating is to gain a realistic understanding of the serving sizes recommended by the CFG. Servings are actually much smaller than most people think, and at this point I would like to give some guidelines as to what constitutes a "serving size." Clearly this matter is somewhat confusing to the patients I counsel. A good understanding of serving sizes helps people determine the minimum amount of food that would be considered adequate for a meal.

What Is a Serving Size?

As I've already mentioned, many women find the CFG scary because they don't believe they can eat the amount of food recommended. In fact, the portions advised are terribly small. It doesn't take much to make a serving. Just having a vegetable in sight on the plate probably constitutes a serving; most people eat double and triple servings and think of them as a single serving. It is a fault of the CFG that serving sizes are not better explained, but of course the CFG is not meant to stand on its own — it is meant to be used as part of a teaching session.

A big problem with the CFG has to do with the number of servings of grain products recommended. The CFG recommends consuming five to twelve of these each day, as it tries to take into account all age and activity groups. I have found that the number twelve is very frightening to the women I counsel and I often put my finger over that number when explaining the CFG. I have also heard the "large" number of grain servings recommended being severely criticized by proponents of low carbohydrate intake. The average woman requires seven to nine servings of grain products a day, depending on her activity level. Two servings of grains then, are roughly equivalent to one-third of the total daily intake of grains recommended by the CFG: remember that I am asking each person to eat about one-third of the day's food at every meal. If you look carefully at serving sizes, you will see that the amount of food involved is not excessive. You may be interested to note that some bagels are so large, they provide five or six grain servings.

Table 2 gives a visual representation of a serving size. I also include, for interest, serving sizes that one might typically be given in a restaurant, where portion sizes seem to be growing and distorting people's understanding of what constitutes proper serving sizes (Table 3). I would also like to mention here that portion sizes in Canada have not yet reached the gargantuan proportions that prevail in the American marketplace.

Table 2: **What Is a Serving?**

	MEASURE	THE SIZE OF . . .
STARCH	1 slice bread	
	1/2 bagel	a hockey puck
	1/2 cup/ 125 mL rice or pasta	a light bulb, small fist or half a baseball
	3/4 cup/ 175 mL hot cereal	fist or cupped hand
	a pancake	a CD
VEGETABLES	1 medium piece	a tennis ball
	1/2 cup/ 125 mL fresh, frozen or canned	a light bulb or small fist
	1 cup/ 250 mL raw greens or salad	a fist or cupped hand
	1/2 cup/ 125 mL tomato sauce	a fried egg
	1/2 cup/ 125 mL broccoli	6 florets
	1 cup/ 250 mL lettuce	4 leaves
	1/2 cup/ 125 mL green beans	8 green beans
FRUITS	1 medium piece	a tennis ball
	1/2 cup/ 125 mL fruit	15 grapes
	1/4 cup/ 50 mL raisins	a large egg
	1/2 cup/ 125 mL melon	8 one-inch/ 2.5 cm cubes
DAIRY	1 cup milk	
	3/4 cup/ 175 mL yogurt	
	1 1/2 oz/ 50 g cheese	2 thumbs, 3 dominoes, a 9-volt battery

PROTEIN	2–3 oz/ 60–90 g meat, poultry or fish	a deck of cards, palm of hand, a computer mouse
	1/2–1 cup/ 125–250 mL beans or lentils	a light bulb or small fist
	2 tbsp/ 30 mL peanut butter	a ping-pong ball
	1–2 eggs	
	4 oz/ 125 g tofu	slightly larger than card deck
OTHER	1/2 cup/ 125 mL ice cream	a tennis ball
	1 pat butter or margarine	a Scrabble tile
	1 tbsp/ 15 mL mayonnaise	a woman's thumb
	1 oz/ 30 g chips or pretzels	2 handfuls

Table 3: Food Guide Serving Sizes Compared to Typical Restaurant Serving Sizes

	FOOD GUIDE SERVING	TYPICAL RESTAURANT SERVING
MEAT	3 oz/ 90 g	6–16 oz/ 180–480 g
SANDWICH	4 oz/ 125 g	9–12 oz/ 270–360 g
PIZZA SLICE	5 oz/ 140 g	9 oz/ 270 g
POPCORN	3 cups/ 750 mL	8–12 cups/ 2–3 L
MUFFIN	2 oz/ 60 g	4 oz/ 125 g
SPAGHETTI WITH TOMATO SAUCE	1 cup/ 250 mL	3 1/2 cups/ 875 mL
FRENCH FRIES	1 1/2 cups/ 375 mL	3 cups/ 750 mL

(Restaurant serving sizes are compiled from information provided by Canada's National Institute of Nutrition, the Washington, DC based Center for Science in the Public Interest, and the University of California at Berkeley Health Letter.)

The Advantages of Structured Eating

The plate method, or circle eating, places a rather strict structure on the day's eating and delivers what I am looking for — three balanced meals throughout the day. Before eating, I want a person to ask, "Is this a meal?" and proceed from there. I hear people say that they "sometimes" have carrot sticks with lunch, or "sometimes" have protein with breakfast or "often" have a sandwich with their salad at lunch. I prefer that they think more in terms of "always" as in, — "I will always seek to eat the components that make up a meal." In the same vein, I don't like the "occasionally" word. The word that I have had on my wall for many years now is that awful word "or" with a line through it. I tell people that I am not the "or" dietitian. I am the "and" dietitian — not cereal or toast but cereal and toast. Not sandwich or salad, but sandwich and salad.

I am not a "take away" dietitian; I seldom tell people what not to eat. I prefer to tell them instead what to eat, because I believe that if we eat three meals a day and include whole grains, whole vegetables and fruits, then we will get sufficient fibre and as a result, will know when to stop eating. In this regard, I'd like to comment on juice — it is a good food, but I would prefer that healthy people get the majority of their vegetables and fruit servings by eating the whole vegetable or fruit. When we chew, rather than drink, our calories, the food we take in will have more of a filling factor.

I find that when people eat in the balanced way I am describing here, they aren't as hungry for junk foods. Also, note that treats can be included in this approach. But I ask people to eat their meals first, and then have dessert. When

I counsel very health-conscious people, I suggest making even treats "count" — cookies can be made with whole wheat flour, oatmeal or raisins, muffins with pineapple, carrots or zucchini. Fruit based desserts also fit well with this approach.

The circle or plate eating structure is firm, but the potential variety within the structure is enormous. Having said this, I realize that unusual things happen to take us away from our routines. I'm asking that in as much as a person can bring regularity to her life, that she include patterns of healthy eating as well.

In fact, my ultimate goal in teaching the circle method is to help my patients simplify and routinize eating habits, so they aren't chores but reflexive acts. In some ways I want eating well to be as easy as brushing one's teeth. Not many people debate with themselves at the end of the day as to whether or not to brush their teeth. I feel it is when we have to think too much about nutrition that feeding ourselves properly becomes difficult. By forming habits, one reduces the need to make too many choices. I'd like to give an example. I happen to live close enough to Health Watch that I can walk to work. When I first realized this I told myself that I would walk home from work three days a week. As a result, every day I had to decide if this would be a walking day or a subway day. It became a burden, in a way, to propel myself toward the back door for my walk home rather than toward the front door and the subway entrance. When I decided to simply walk home every day, my feet just naturally took the back route out of the building. I no longer had to debate about what I "should" do. I want nutrition to be like that. Why should people have to decide over and over again whether to eat a treat or have something healthy? I want people to think of healthy food as being both their routine food and a treat.

My experience with my patients has borne out my belief that following the plate or circle method of eating, that is, simply glancing at each meal plate to see if it satisfies the definition of a meal, makes it much easier to eat a healthy diet. I don't believe that achieving good nutrition has to be complicated or confusing — I believe that it can be basic and simple. Of course, there is room for fine tuning, for adjusting according to individual requirements or even for weight loss. But the basic foundation of a healthy total eating pattern needs to be in place before fine tuning can be effective.

The Fatigue-Fighter Plan

Another approach to circle eating is the "Fatigue-Fighter Plan" that my colleague Andrea Miller and I devised together. Andrea and I created the Fatigue-Fighter Plan in response to our observation that people are drawn to diets. Regular, everyday eating cannot compete, we noticed, with anything that sounds the teeniest bit interesting (read complicated). Perhaps the degree of difficulty enhances a diet's desirability! In any case, if diets appeal to you, then here is one that puts the plate method into action and is nourishing. The Fatigue-Fighter Plan is unlike most diets, though, in that people are able to stay on it.

The Fatigue-Fighter Plan

TIMING IS ESSENTIAL
• Eat within the first hour of waking.
• All day long, do not go longer than 3 to 4 hours without eating.

FOCUS ON MEALS
• Eat at least 3 meals a day.
• Eat 1 to 2 snacks a day.

WHAT IS A MEAL?

Meals must include:	For example ...
Protein	Meat, fish, poultry, beans, tofu, cheese, eggs, nuts, seeds
PLUS **Starch**	Rice, pasta, potato, bread, cereal, oats, quinoa, millet
PLUS **Vegetables**	Spinach, kale, squash, broccoli, carrots, onions, garlic, tomatoes
PLUS **Fruit**	Melons, kiwi, berries, oranges
PLUS **Calcium** source	Milk, cheese, yogurt, enriched soy or rice milk, enriched orange juice, tofu
PLUS **Fats and Oils**	Nuts, seeds, flaxseed, canola oil, olive oil, sesame oil, avocado

Normal Eating

Over time, circle eating or following the Fatigue-Fighter Plan helps us re-establish normal eating patterns. Left to their own devices, our bodies know how to nourish themselves. When we heed our body's signals, without getting caught up in guilt or worry, we eat normally. Many of the women who come to Health Watch already know how to eat a healthy diet and how to eat normally. A definition of normal eating that I particularly like comes from Ellyn Satter's book, *Secrets of Feeding a Healthy Family* (Madison, WI: Kelcy Press, 1999):

> Normal eating is going to the table hungry and eating until you are satisfied ... It is being able to choose food you like and eat it and truly get enough of it, not just stop eating because you think you should. Normal eating is being able to give some thought to your food selection so you get nutritious food, but not being so wary and restrictive that you miss out on enjoyable food. Normal eating is giving yourself permission to eat sometimes because you are happy, sad or bored, or just because it feels good. Normal eating is three meals a day, or four or five, or it can be choosing to munch along the way. It is leaving some cookies on the plate because you know you can have some again tomorrow, or it is eating more now because they taste so wonderful. Normal eating is overeating at times and wishing you had more. Normal eating is trusting your body to make up for your mistakes in eating. Normal eating takes up some of your time and attention, but keeps its place as only one important area of your life. In short, normal eating is flexible. It varies in response to your hunger, your schedule, your proximity to food and your feelings. (p. 5)

My patient Stephanie echoes Satter's balanced, guilt-free attitude to food and eating:

> It's important to eat proper food but a little
> junk food I don't feel really hurts you. You
> can't just eat healthy food and nothing else
> unless you are so geared to that that it would
> bother you to have something. I love salt, I
> love sweet things and I have some of it when
> I crave it. Do it now and again so that you
> don't feel deprived.
>
> STEPHANIE, 49

When we eat normally, we respect our appetite. We know that appetite and hunger are not our enemies, but that appetite is a sign of health. It is our body's way of saying, "I'm ready for some food." Without food we die. "I work in a hospital," I often tell people. "In a hospital," I explain, "the value of appetite becomes very clear. When the very old and the very sick lose their appetites, it often appears that that is one way in which they are preparing to go." But what about experiencing increased appetite as a result of eating more? This is a worry my patients express again and again. I tell people to go ahead and eat — "Your body is having a party," I say. "It did not think you were listening before when it told you it was hungry. To not feel hunger when you have not eaten is what is abnormal. So trust your hunger. Eventually it will calm down. Choose your foods wisely, and make sure there is plenty of fibre in what you eat. If you feel that you have overeaten when you reach the end of the day, then go lightly at supper. But if you have done it the other way around, if you have eaten lightly all day, then there is no way to stop eating at night. You are sliding down that hill with no brakes."

Having said this, I believe that for most people there comes a point in life where one has to choose between normal eating and weight. That is, in order to occasionally eat dessert, one may have to be content with a few extra pounds. Clearly, some women are not prepared to jeopardize their weight in any way. In fact, one of my patients, an unnaturally thin woman who works as a model, could not even consider eating normally, knowing she would surely start to gain weight if she did. But one wise woman, after expressing the view that perhaps she should lose weight, and then hearing me respond with concern that she would soon reach the age at which weight naturally starts to decline (about seventy), sighed with relief. "I didn't really want to give up my treats, anyway," she said.

Sometimes I wish I could harness all the energy that women put into worrying about their weight and dieting, because that would be a powerful force we could apply to something that could truly affect the world in a positive way. That said, let's now look at the question of weight loss.

3

Diets, Weight Loss
and Healthy Eating

When I first started working at Health Watch, weighing of patients was a routine part of a visit with me and the scale was the first thing women saw as they walked into my office. I soon noticed the extreme apprehension patients had as they walked through my door to face the scale. Some women would start to disrobe before the door was even closed, removing jewellery and in one case, a heavy leather skirt. I'm sure some women experienced elevated blood pressure as they prepared to be weighed. The medical director was very sympathetic to my request to discontinue routine weighing of patients. But when I just ignored the scale I could see some people thinking they were somehow getting away with not being weighed. The apprehension remained until I moved the scale to the back of the office and hung some posters on it to make it more attractive. Why haven't I removed it altogether? Some people, for reasons of their own, want to be weighed, and I want to be able to weigh them when I am concerned that people are experiencing an unhealthy weight loss. In general, however, weighing my patients, I maintain, distracts them from what is really important. I want people to focus on increasing their activity and eating healthy food, not on weight loss diets, which have such a bad track record. Health benefits generally result from positive changes in activity and diet, regardless of whether or not weight is lost. The point was well made in May 2000, when the theme of Healthy Weight week, a week promoted and sponsored by the Healthy Weight Network was "Lose weight — throw away your scale." (For more information on the Healthy Weight network, see "Internet Resources," p. 160.)

How and Why Diets Don't Work

I said above that diets have a poor track record. I'd like to discuss active dieting. So far I have been talking about triangle eating — people following this pattern eat less during the day when they are less likely to notice their hunger and then succumb to heavier eating in the evening. An active dieter will eat lightly throughout the entire day, with no binges occurring. The dieter is usually following a prescribed meal plan found in a magazine or book or which was given to her by a dieting centre.

My patients try all kinds of diets, and diet fashions, like clothing fashions, are always changing. Three decades ago we were first introduced to the low-carbohydrate approach to weight loss, which after a few years went out of style. In fact, when I first started working at Health Watch I could almost guess a person's age based on whether or not they believed that bread was fattening. The low-carbohydrate fad has now returned with a vengeance. But we also have Weight Watchers, Herbal Magic, Dr. Bernstein, Suzanne Somers, with her emphasis on food combining (or not combining, as the case may be) and so on. There are a number of scientific journal articles pointing out that what all the diets promoted by these authorities have in common is that they are low in calories.

Now I was taught in my nutrition course at university that in order to lose weight a person has to cut calories. I was shown how to calculate energy intake and needs and then to subtract 500 or 1,000 calories from these amounts to achieve a slow progressive weight loss. It is well understood that for most people the strategy works, at least in the short term. So when people tell me how much their neighbour or sister or workmate lost on such and such a diet, I am not impressed. Losing weight is not the difficult part. The difficult part is keeping it off, and this is where I believe that all diets fail because no diet can be followed indefinitely. Permanent weight loss occurs not from dieting, but from changing over to a new, healthier way of eating.

To me, dieting is another version of triangle eating, one that occurs over a longer time period. The beginning days of the diet can be thought of as the top of the triangle. The dieter is feeling good about her weight loss and doesn't really notice her hunger. But by the four o'clock point in the triangle eater's day, corresponding to weeks or months into a diet, the dieter is starting to notice how hungry she really is. By eight in the evening of the triangle, corresponding to that point when the dieter cannot tolerate a fuel shortage any longer, the binge eating begins. The diet has failed to provide enough food to supply fuel requirements and the person has to eat to catch up. Weight is regained.

A Dietitian Challenged by Diets

Even though diets don't work, I'm no longer surprised that so many of my patients follow them. The most common concern my patients express is that they are overweight. Much as I try to take the emphasis away from weight and towards healthy habits, the desire to look slim is what seems to rule us. My position is that non-age-related weight gain is a symptom of poor health habits — a lack of activity (probably the most important factor) and poor eating habits. One of my patients once referred to weight gain as a barometer of her health; rising weight signalled her to take notice that something was going wrong. I've also noted a statement often made by patients who come to the clinic in the spring. "I've gained some weight over the winter," they say. "I'm not as active in the winter." (They have identified the correct health activity that is at fault.) "So, I've decided to go on a diet," they continue. (I cringe.)

But I wonder if I am wrong not to pay more attention to weight. After all, concern about weight is usually what motivates people to start eating a more healthy diet in the first place. I particularly have difficulty being as supportive as I want to be to those patients who come in reporting weight loss — I tend to focus on the shortfalls of their diet rather than on their weight loss accomplishment. I am trying to learn how to celebrate these women's achievements with them, and at the same time communicate the pitfalls I see ahead.

"I've lost fifteen pounds and I've been on a diet for five months," a woman will say. I look at the diet section of her Health Watch form and see how she's eating. I've tried to discourage further dieting, but my words have fallen on deaf ears, as the woman has the proof of her success. What I see is that she is underfuelling her body and that at some point she will start eating again and the weight will return, which, of course, is how most weight loss efforts end. "Let's see how you can maintain that weight loss. Are you hungry?" I ask. "Because if you aren't now, you probably will be. Let me explain what to do when you notice that you are starting to get cravings, when your body starts to tell you that it is hungry and would like to start getting its required number of calories for the day." And that's when I launch into my "eat meal foods and practise rectangle eating" message.

I might also remind her that research evidence shows that people can achieve such health goals as lowered blood pressure, cholesterol, and blood sugar by eating and exercising in a healthy way, even if they achieve no weight loss with the new healthier pattern. Of course, diets can sometimes be the ally of healthy eating habits. I often ask people how they are eating differently now that they're on a diet. "I cut out the junk," they say. Other common statements include: "I eat breakfast," "I'm having protein with my meals," and "I'm eating more vegetables and fruit."

I am left wondering why a diet was necessary for these healthy changes to be made. So I sometimes ask people directly, "Why didn't you do this last year, when I told you the same things? Why do you need a diet to do these things?" My patients reply that they need a structure, some accounting to someone else, some motivation to keep on track. And so I am trying to be more accepting of their emphasis on weight loss. I still don't understand why people prefer some complicated pattern of eating in order to change their habits, though. Why should normal, balanced, healthy eating be so boring? I haven't figured that one out yet, which is why I must continue to explore the question with my patients at Health Watch.

Don't Be Fooled by "Diet Magic"

Several things about common approaches to dieting also trigger knee-jerk responses in me. When I see some foods on the diet history, I feel very uncomfortable — melba toast, cottage cheese, and Special K, for example. I believe these foods are traditional diet foods and I often make a point of asking people if they like these foods. (I think the reason I ask is because years ago a woman told me that she had to eat fish three times a week on her weight loss diet and she hated fish!) Patients usually reply that they do like these foods, but I still feel that they eat them because they believe they are less fattening. Another thing on the history that makes me uncomfortable are supplements people take to suppress their appetites, including chromium, apple cider vinegar capsules, and certain herbal supplements. Some diets rely on the appetite suppressant ephedra, whose safety is under review. On other histories I'll note that the woman is not eating certain foods at the same time, in the belief that this will trick her metabolism into burning food more efficiently.

When I see these things on a history, I explain that there is no magic in foods. Diet foods do not cause weight loss and you don't have to eat them if you don't want to. Special

K may taste good but it contains the same number of calories as any other plain cereal, and lacks the fibre of a whole grain cereal, I might add. Melba toast is tasty. But there is nothing special about its ability to cause weight loss other than that the dieter just eats a few pieces at a time and therefore takes in fewer calories than if she had a slice of bread. Whenever I see melba toast, or Hollywood or Weight Watcher's bread (breads sliced so thinly that one slice is equivalent to one-half slice of regular bread) on a diet history, I explain that the main effect these foods have is to make us hungry — they provide too few calories to prevent later binge eating in the evening. There is no pill that will melt fat. Chromium will not take away your appetite — and why are you trying to take away your appetite in the first place? I believe in being thankful for appetite because it is a sign that we are healthy and alive. Night appetite, as I've tried to show, simply means that you haven't had enough food during the day.

As for food combining, Suzanne Somers has yet to convince me of its worth. To me it just adds an unnecessary degree of complexity to the day. In Suzanne Somers' plan the dieter is told not to eat protein and starch at the same meal. I believe that this way of eating is counter to the way most people eat and awkward to explain to one's host when invited out to a meal. More importantly, I believe it's difficult enough just to eat three balanced meals a day, much less to have to wade through complicated food rituals. Some people have no trouble eating these major food categories separately. But I have seen those who will eat protein at meals and forget to eat the starch. One woman I saw who was trying to follow a food combining diet ate only starch with her meals and forgot to eat any protein at all!

I repeat, there is no magic to weight loss. To lose weight you have to exercise and you have to eat in a balanced way, to provide your body with nutrients and avoid creating the ravenous hunger that leads to binge eating. Of course, you can choose lower-calorie versions of your favourite foods, eat fewer portions and eliminate any extras, and this will facilitate your weight loss. I put a lot of emphasis on foods high in fibre since these tend to be low in calories, high in nutrients, and filling, helping to satisfy hunger. Keep in mind too that it is very easy to drink calories in the form of pop, alcoholic beverages and even juice, and not even be aware you've had anything to "eat." And I have pretty well decided that to lose weight after the age of forty, you have to be super vigilant and allow no "extras" or "treats" that add calories to your diet.

Diet — Belittling and Disrespectful

I must conclude this chapter by admitting there's a deeper reason I dislike diets so much. It's not just that I believe that diets don't work, and that they may, in fact, cause weight gain. I dislike diets because I believe they are belittling and disrespectful. The diet says, "You don't get to eat normally, you can't have a whole sandwich, you can only eat half a banana." What is the woman who doesn't eat breakfast saying about herself to the rest of the family? I was intrigued by one patient who ate three-quarters of a sandwich at lunch. She was too hungry to eat only half, but knew that a whole sandwich would surely make her fat and so she compromised. In my view, the act of eating less than a normal serving size, of not allowing oneself to eat a whole sandwich, sends the message that one is less of a person.

And what does everyone think when they start bingeing? In the afternoon, eating is called cheating. At night, the recriminations begin: "What's the matter with me? Why do I have no self control? I'm a failure!" What do I think? I think you know by now: "You haven't had enough fuel in your day, you're just hungry." I really dislike that "cheat" word as you can well imagine. I once read a wonderful quote in a woman's magazine from Emme, a plus size model. She said, "If you cheat on your husband, that's bad. But a cookie is just a cookie."

Will eating the way I advocate always cause weight loss? I don't know. I don't have an absolute answer for weight loss or else, as I tell my patients, I would not be here right now. I would, instead, be the richest person in the world. If you have gained weight because of unhealthy eating or more probably because of low physical activity, then yes, I believe weight loss is possible if you change your habits. But my emphasis is always on health and healthy habits because I know those are destined to be beneficial, whether or not weight loss occurs. I am also certain that triangle eating does not cause weight loss and may cause weight gain, so why not stick to rectangle eating? As with triangle eating, you may not lose weight, but you will be better fuelled and better nourished.

And is everyone meant to lose weight, I wonder? One of my patients told me that she was like a St. Bernard dog, and she had no interest in being, nor could she ever be, a chihuahua! We come in all shapes and sizes; the goal I advocate is health at every size.

4

Carbohydrate, Fat, Calcium and Vitamins

I've now made a number of references to starch, carbohydrates and fat. Starches are carbohydrates and the two words are often used interchangeably. Starch, carbohydrates and fat are "charged" words. Each creates a unique image in a person's mind. Some people love starchy foods. Some people fear them, because of the association that has been created between starch intake and weight gain. Some people love white, crusty bread. Others prefer whole grain products. A nutrition message that has become "stuck" in people's minds is that "fat is bad." I have come to believe that this idea is not necessarily true. At the very least, the matter is not so simple. Nutrition messages can and do change and this can be very confusing for people, me included. But I believe that by sticking to nutrition basics, as I have already outlined, one can achieve nutritious eating and better health without falling victim to changing nutrition fashions. I would like to share with you what I tell my patients about carbohydrates and fat. I also include a section on calcium, as well as a section on why I believe that taking a multivitamin-mineral supplement is a good thing to do.

Carbohydrate

Carbohydrate foods supply essential nutrients, including protein and fibre, and serve as a primary source of fuel. Carbohydrates can be starches, as found in grain foods, legumes, potatoes and other starchy vegetables like carrots, or carbohydrates can be sugars, found in fruit, juice or milk. (Sugars are also eaten as sugars, on their own or in foods.) Unfortunately, the idea that one's diet should be low in carbohydrate has permeated everyday thought. I was once having a discussion with a nursing friend about vitamins. A nearby student doctor was eavesdropping. He didn't believe in taking vitamins and that made all my opinions suspect. He expressed his displeasure by muttering, "And who could ever eat twelve servings of carb a day?" (This is the largest number of servings of grain products suggested by Canada's Food Guide.) He was implying, I believe, that I could not possibly know anything, that I was a stupid dietitian who believed in the Food Guide. "I'm on the high protein diet and I lost twenty pounds," he added. He's not alone in his view. Many of my patients believe carbs are bad for them, that they make a person fat. I had one patient who, after I eloquently, I believed, explained that her carbohydrate craving was actually a craving for fat, told me that if it weren't for the bread, she wouldn't be eating all that fatty cheese. In her mind, bread really was the problem.

I do not want to get into a discussion about carbohydrate nutrition. It is impossible to eat a diet free of carbohydrates nor should we want to. The question becomes, are we eating too much carbohydrate? I believe that this only became an important question when dieting gurus began associating eating too much carbohydrate with gaining weight. Their assertion has never been proven. Carbohydrates do supply fuel, and when fuel consumption exceeds fuel expenditure, people gain weight. I don't believe that carbohydrates have a particular penchant for causing weight gain, that there is something inherent in their make-up that causes them to be fattening. For the majority of the world's populations, carbohydrates are the dietary staple. If you were to overeat carbohydrate, then yes, you would probably gain weight. I believe that carbohydrates eaten in the context of a balanced diet, however, contribute to our health and do not cause weight gain.

This possibility is summarized in a review, *Grains in the Canadian Diet* prepared by Canada's National Institute of Nutrition and published in 1999:

> High carbohydrate, high fibre diets appear to be associated with lower energy intakes and lower body weight, both over the short and the long term. The main mechanisms seem to be the lower energy density of these diets and their effect on satiety. Most grain products, being of low energy density and high in carbohydrate and fibre, would appear to contribute to the maintenance of optimum body weight.

I believe that if we want to lose weight we can easily eliminate sugar and high calorie carbohydrate sweets and desserts. But I see what happens when people eliminate the carbohydrate portion of their breakfasts and lunches — they binge on cookies! Low carbohydrate diets in general lack variety and interest and ultimately become monotonous. Some of these diets are so strict that the dieter is not "allowed" to eat favourite foods such as bananas or carrots, since they are considered to be too high in carbohydrate. But as these diets do nothing to address basic unbalanced eating habits, the low carbohydrate dieter, like any other dieter, regains the lost weight when previous eating habits are resumed, as inevitably happens.

Some women tell me that when they reduce their consumption of bread they feel less bloated. I do not think these people have to cut out all carbohydrates, but I pay attention to what they are telling me. I ask them to consider that they may be reacting to the particular grain that the bread they eat is made from and that it may be worthwhile for them to experiment with other grains. "Don't throw the baby out with the bath water," I say. That is, if wheat is the problem, don't stop eating all grains. Switch to rice, oats, quinoa and millet.

Fat

Of all the nutrition messages that health professionals have broadcast over the years, none has stuck in people's minds quite as thoroughly as the "fat is bad" one. I have had patients who eat practically no fat at all. People routinely cut red meat from their diets, eschew butter, banish avocado, and cook with only small amounts of oil, in the interests not only of weight loss, but of health. But the "fat is bad" message is presently being reworked. In a fascinating article published in *Science Magazine* in March 2001, Gary Taubes convincingly presents the argument that there is no real scientific proof that high fat diets cause heart disease or cancer. I believe that the issue is becoming one not of how much fat is in the diet, but what kind. There is growing evidence that the types of fat found in fatty fish (salmon, mackerel and sardines for example) are extremely beneficial to health, and nuts have joined the ranks of "health" foods for the fat, fibre and other nutrients they contain. Unfortunately people who are dieting generally end up cutting out food sources of these healthy fats but are more likely to binge on high fat snacks that don't, however, contain healthy fats.

It is true that fat and fatty foods have more calories, as I've already mentioned. They are what is called calorie dense. That is why hungry people reach for them when they are bingeing. But if you regularly eat the foods recommended by the Food Guide, including high fibre grains, vegetables and fruits, then you will not have to struggle with cravings for high fat snack foods. If you are watching your weight, then limit, but do not cut out, fatty foods. Focus on the fats and fatty foods that have been found to be healthy: olive and canola oil, ground flax seeds and flax oil, fatty fish and nuts.

Calcium

One nutrient I focus on at Health Watch is calcium. I think that part of the reason dietitians pay attention to calcium is because it is one nutrient that we know a lot about. Calcium is important not only for bone health — it plays a role in maintaining healthy blood pressure and in controlling PMS symptoms. It can be obtained in sufficient amounts mainly from one food group, dairy, and, although there are books available telling us how to meet our calcium needs without eating dairy foods, I don't believe doing so is possible or practical for most people. Nowadays there are also calcium-fortified foods available, including soy and rice beverages and orange juice. I personally do not see much difference between drinking orange juice enriched with calcium and taking a calcium pill with water, but I try to take people's preferences into account. Someone who hates taking pills and drinks a cup of orange juice on a daily basis, for example, would clearly be more likely to get their needed calcium from fortified juice than from a supplement. Essentially my personal approach is to make getting enough calcium as practical as possible for my patients, and to help them make sure that they consume the required amount, not occasionally, but every day. I determine how much dairy a person is able and willing to consume (for I do acknowledge that not everyone is meant to consume dairy products), subtract the calcium obtained from the amount required daily, and supplement the rest in one form or another. It is because of calcium's importance to health that the Fatigue-Fighter Plan outlined in chapter 2 includes a serving of calcium-rich food (or a supplement) at each meal, as an essential part of a balanced meal.

Multivitamin-Mineral Supplements

I am not alone in thinking that most people would benefit from taking a multivitamin-mineral supplement. In an article published in the prestigious *New England Journal of Medicine* in December 2001, two eminent American nutritionists argue that there is substantial evidence supporting a beneficial role for higher intakes of folic acid, vitamin B6, vitamin B12 and vitamin D for many people and they believe that a basic multivitamin will ensure an adequate intake of other vitamins for which the evidence of benefit is indirect. The people they identify as those for whom a multivitamin would be especially important are women who might become pregnant, persons who regularly consume one or two alcoholic drinks per day, the elderly, vegans and people not able to consume sufficient vegetables and fruit.

With my patients, I equate taking a multivitamin-mineral supplement to taking out insurance on a house or car. To me a multivitamin-mineral is nutritional insurance, meant to fill any gaps that might arise from time to time in a healthy balanced diet.

I have given you my perspective on health issues that I deal with on a daily basis. Not everybody agrees with me, nor, in fact, should they — I don't have a licence on knowledge. I also realize that people can achieve health through many actions other than eating a balanced diet and taking vitamins. Before I talk about what the women of Health Watch have taught me about that, I would like to explain what I see as the barriers to good nutrition.

5

Overcoming Barriers to Good Nutrition

Ask the average person what the constituents of a healthy diet are and you will hear responses such as low fat, lots of vegetables and fruits, less meat. The nutrition message, despite sometimes being contradictory or confusing in the media, has gotten through. We all know good nutrition is important. But do most people eat in the way they know is best? In my experience, no. Why not? I think three factors interfere with people's ability to eat in a healthy way: lack of time, the pressure to be thin and the inability to apply knowledge to themselves. I would like to talk about each of these factors separately to point out how they might intermingle to reinforce each other, and, most importantly, to look at how they can be overcome.

Lack of Time
The first and foremost factor in daily life that influences how a person eats is time. I read recently that we live in a

time famine. Indeed, nobody seems to have time for anything except work. As a result, we often skip meals, and the meal we most often sacrifice is breakfast. We leave the house in the morning without having had any food or we eat breakfast in the car. Dashboard dining is now so common that it has generated equipment to go with it: those cups and plates that can be affixed to the inside of a moving vehicle so they don't topple. I saw an interesting variation on dashboard dining one day on my way to work — a person riding a bicycle with a bun in one hand and a cup of something in the other. This intrepid cyclist alternately raised one hand and then the other to the mouth and back to the handlebars. Handlebar dining!

We eat lunch at our desks (this is called having a lap lunch) or we skip lunch altogether. We pick up supper on the way home from work, or we may not have time for supper if we work late or go to the fitness club.

Remember that food is fuel. When there is a fuel deficit, there is an energy deficit. Just as a car needs fuel to go, so do we need food. We know that we cannot delay the filling of our car's gas tank, yet we fail to pay attention to our own fuel needs. When it is time to get more gas, people don't throw their arms up in the air and moan, "I don't have time to get more gas!" Yet, people are continually frustrated by the time it takes not only to prepare a meal, but to eat it. We also know that if it takes a full tank of gas to drive to somewhere, let's say to Health Watch, we cannot expect our car to take us there on a mere teaspoon, even if we perhaps stop for another teaspoon of fuel along the way. Yet, in our quest to save time, we routinely push our bodies to meet our goals on the equivalent of mere teaspoons of fuel.

What are the consequences of this way of life? First and foremost, we are not as healthy as we could be. Meals are the main occasions at which we eat whole grains and vegetables, the foods that provide the nourishment our bodies need, and the first foods to disappear when we insist we have no time. I see that people who eat more regularly have more energy and feel better. I also see that when people eat fewer plant foods, especially during the critical hours of the working day, they tend to succumb to poorer quality food later in the day. Think back to that car: when it is time to refuel we don't say, "I don't have time to go to the gas station! I'll just stop at the side of the road and throw in some sand and gravel. That will keep the car going until the end of the day." Of course not. Yet we continually become irritated by the idea of stopping what we're doing to fuel our bodies and when we are finally forced to stop because if we don't we'll faint, we throw the equivalent of sand and gravel into our stomachs.

Not only the nutritional quality of food is compromised by our fast paced no-time-for-meals lifestyle. We are also experiencing the decline of the family meal. A recent study, published in the *Archives of Family Medicine* in March 2000, reports that the percentage of American families who regularly eat together has been steadily declining. The researchers found that women in their sixties and seventies remember eating together with their family 97 to 98 percent of the time when they were children; today only 43 percent of the nine- to fourteen-year-old children studied ate dinner with their family every day. The study also reports that a phone survey of parents of twelve- to seventeen-year-olds indicated that only 27 percent of these teens ate dinner together with their family every day. The study goes on to suggest that an association exists between the frequency of family dinners and the nutritional quality of children's diets. The more a family eats together, the researchers found, the higher was each member's consumption of fruits and vegetables and several beneficial nutrients.

Unfortunately it is often only when women approach menopause that they begin to take care of themselves; this is especially true of married women. The children are grown enough or gone and there is more time for "me." It is often also at this age that women begin to come to Health Watch. These are the women who have been preparing nutritious meals for their families, making their children eat breakfast and packing their lunches. They may have devoted a lot of energy to their jobs. And they are likely the same women who have been missing breakfast and scrabbling for enough food during the day.

Overcoming the Time Barrier

My patient Diana, 40, commented to me once, "Everyone has become so busy they feel they don't have time for health, but the fact of the matter is that if they would set aside the time they would actually find that their whole day would be better." If her words make sense to you, I encourage you to let them inspire you to develop strategies for overcoming the time barrier.

People skip breakfast because they don't want to get up earlier. People skip lunch because they don't stop working. I sometimes ask my patients to make appointments with themselves for lunch so that they will be forced to stop working.

Many of our patients at Health Watch are teachers. Many of these teachers rarely eat lunch, due to the fact that they are spending their lunch hours with students. Much as I might appreciate their sacrifice were I the parent of some of these students, I am not happy as their dietitian. The "no lunch" attitude is common in many professions and I do my best to change it. To me, the words "I don't have time" really mean, "I don't take the time." Now to be honest, I have talked to some people who really are given no breaks during their work day. One woman, in charge of reception and switchboard at a busy company, explained that she receives little relief for washroom breaks, let alone time off to eat lunch. People in service industries are frequently victims of their clientele. One woman, a hairstylist, complained to me that people regularly entered her private area, which is behind a curtain and marked "Private."

But even if this is your situation, you can still start the day with breakfast. This is a meal over which everyone has control. It doesn't take long to make breakfast, say to slap two pieces of whole wheat bread around some peanut butter and grab a banana. You can take such a simple meal with you, get to work ten minutes early, and eat it there. My colleague Andrea Miller tells her patients to take the time to have cereal. She says it takes two bites to get through two pieces of toast, but when you chew your way through cereal you not only get some calcium from the milk you add to it, you feel as if you've had a substantial amount of food. And the fact is, cereal is more filling. Slice a banana into the bowl to keep your meal balanced and in line with "circle eating." Once they're on the job, I tell my patients to assert to themselves that their well-being is worth taking the time needed to eat. Stopping work at lunch-time to eat a healthy meal can only have positive results. The break helps us to relax, refuel, perhaps take a walk and ultimately return to work refreshed and better able to get the task done than if no break is taken at all.

Not that eating a meal has to take a lot of time — you can eat lunch at your desk if you have to. Just make sure you've got your protein, your starch, your vegetables and your fruit. If you can't eat all of it, save the rest for later. You can pack your lunch (try cooking extra at dinner and setting it aside), you can carry parts of it (the vegetables and fruit, for example), you can buy it or you can keep supplies at work. What I often say is that your food, unlike your outfit, doesn't have to match. Food doesn't have to be specially cooked, it doesn't have to be fancy — it just has to be balanced.

The Pressure To Be Thin

A second factor that interferes with good nutrition is the pressure to be thin. I believe that we live in a time of disdain for the average female body. How else can we explain the constant attacks that both the media and individuals make on women's body sizes and the social expectations that we shrink to an impossible size and shape? The woman held up today as the image of beauty is perhaps half the size of the desirable woman of a few decades ago. While shopping with my daughter one day I noticed how tiny the clothing on display was. I knew I could never squeeze into such skimpy pants. (Fortunately my daughter also understood that she couldn't, and she didn't let the fact bother her.) A discussion of how women are encouraged to manipulate their bodies in

order to achieve looks that are in line with popular defini-
tions of beauty is beyond the scope of what I want to discuss
here. Besides, I like to believe that we have gone as far as we
can in our attempts to shrink the female body and that we
will soon reverse course and start appreciating once more a
realistic, healthy size. My patient Susan, 49, is a harbinger of
this attitude when she says,

> I think a person is attractive if they're com-
> fortable with themselves. There's something
> about confidence and how you carry your-
> self that makes you attractive. Some people
> are meant to be slim and they're attractive
> because they're comfortable with that. I'm
> five foot one inch and I've always been ten
> pounds overweight. But I also think I'm a
> reasonably attractive, comfortable looking
> person.

Unfortunately, not everyone is as comfortable with their
size as Susan is. The pressure to be thin that women
encounter on a daily basis instills in many of my patients a
terrible fear of getting fat, since weight gain becomes associated with failure and social and romantic rejection. In the
face of this fear, people rationalize skipping meals because
they believe that by consuming fewer calories they will lose
weight. Many women I see have been dieting for a large portion of their lives and have learned how to successfully get
through the day with a minimum of food. They equate
being "good" with not eating and being "bad" with giving in
to their hunger. They feel a sense of achievement in "win-

ning," that is, going through long periods of not eating. In fact, many such women have divorced themselves from their natural hunger to the point that they no longer recognize it. I have had women tell me they never get hungry, and then relate that sometimes they feel faint or shaky. One young woman who visited me was puzzled by the fact that she sometimes had a growling stomach — she had never learned that her stomach's sounds are a primary hunger signal. Many chronic dieters are terrified to eat an adequate breakfast because doing so triggers a hunger they don't have if they skip breakfast. They believe that if they have breakfast, they will then eat all day in the same compulsive, hungry way they do at night. They have come to believe that bingeing at night is normal and something they will always do. I don't dwell on the scientific reason for the increased appetite that accompanies breakfast; instead, I remind my patients that by eating early in the day they will normalize their bodies' appetite mechanism and that normal appetite is a sign of health. And I reassure them that eating more nutritious food during the day will lead to less eating in the evening.

For those trying desperately to please the social conventions that barrage women with the message to be thin, food, hunger and appetite have all become the enemy. Not only do women who are trying to be thin see stopping to eat food as an annoyance in the middle of a busy day, they see food as containing calories, the biggest enemy of all, because calories, in turn, represent weight gain. (However, it seems to be only the calories consumed at breakfast and lunch that "count." Calories eaten at other times seem not to "count," in fact, they may not even be remembered.) As a result of the desire to avoid calories, the precursor of food consumption, appetite, is avoided at all costs by some of my patients. Women try to suppress hunger by drinking copious amounts of water or coffee. I refer to these strategies as trying to drown appetite, in the case of water consumption, or to drug it into oblivion, in the case of caffeine use. Women will also try to eat as little as possible. "I can't eat that much breakfast or else I'm starving an hour later!" is what I very often hear. People can more easily skip daytime meals and mask normal daytime hunger — they are too busy to notice their fuel shortage. Come evening, however, hunger takes control. Hunger, not boredom, lack of will-power or weakness of character makes women eat. In the end, none of the methods for suppressing and ignoring hunger work, simply because the body needs to replenish its energy stores sooner or later. What's more, there is no benefit, as already discussed, in delayed eating.

As also discussed earlier, in order to cut out calories women cut out meals during the day and thereby reduce their consumption of vegetables and whole grains, the "meal foods" that deliver nutrients. They also reduce their consumption of fibre (found only in plant foods), a food component that plays a key role in the health of our digestive tract and helps lower cholesterol levels. They reduce their intake of phytochemicals, those components of plant foods that have widespread beneficial health effects. They drink less milk because it has too many calories and compromise their calcium status, as they don't always replace the milk with supplements. Finally, they increase their evening consumption of poor quality fuel in their attempts finally to fill up — eating the equivalent of sand and gravel. And, as I discussed in the chapter on triangle eating, people who skip and skimp on meals in order to lose weight, are, I believe, on a weight gain regimen. In other words, diets cause weight gain, because even people who can "diet" all day inevitably eat at night. They then tend to choose more calorie-dense foods and consume them at a time when storage is favoured over metabolism.

My patient, Alicia, 35, gives a good description of what I have been saying:

> Picture an animal in a forest not getting any food for two weeks. Its metabolism will slow down, it'll lose a little bit of weight, it'll slow down and won't have as much energy. Then when it catches an animal it'll eat the whole thing and the body will store the fat and store all the nutrients because it doesn't know when the animal's going to get fed again. The human body works the same. It doesn't know when it's going to get fed again so it will store everything you give it after this foolish diet and therefore you'll gain twice as much, maybe more, weight back.

Health Watch women, like all women, struggle with their body image. They do not always accept my interpretation of how their diets sabotage their health and even their weight goals. In addition, many of the women who come are in the menopausal age range. Menopause is often accompanied by weight gain, whether due to decreased activity as we get older, the decreased metabolism that comes with ageing, or decreased hormone levels. Women who have seldom given thought to their weight before all of a sudden realize they have a "tummy" to contend with — weight tends to accumulate in the waist and stomach area at this age. I've tried to liken this stomach to a badge of membership in the menopause club, equating it with a desirable and enviable stage in a woman's life. The Mayo Clinic tells women to get used to their increased waistline and the December 1998 *Mayo Clinic Woman's Health Source* letter tells women to "get out and buy another pair of jeans." I'm not even sure how judgemental women are towards others' stomachs. One thing I have noticed, however, is that women are always skinnier on the other side of the room. And by extension everyone assumes that I, too, must have a smaller tummy, I who sit on the other side of the table.

In her book, *The Change Before the Change: Everything You Need to Know to Stay Healthy in the Decade Before Menopause* (New York: Bantam Doubleday Dell, 2000), Laura Corio explains that women's bodies change in shape around menopause even if there is no weight gain. She states that there is a shifting of weight from the hips and thighs to the belly and breasts: after menopause only 40 percent of women retain their waistline. She attributes this change in fat distribution to a shift in hormones; estrogen predisposes women to break down fat in the abdominal region of the body and store it in the lower body. As estrogen diminishes, the reverse happens. As well, as estrogen decreases, other, androgenic, hormones come to dominate — these hormones stimulate fat accumulation in the abdominal area of the body.

There may be some confusion here between menopausal weight gain and shape shifting and the type of weight gain that creates the "apple-shaped" body associated with a higher risk of heart disease. My position is that some weight gain at menopause is normal and natural and that it can be contained by a commitment to healthy eating and exercise habits. I do not want to imply that I am complacent about weight and weight gain. My thesis is that people come in all shapes and sizes, and that one must distinguish between weight that is inherited and weight that is a product of unhealthy living.

I see something very self-demeaning in women's pursuit of unnatural thinness — the goal of dieting, after all, is to reduce one's body size. The goal behind healthy eating is to work towards being as healthy as one can be at any weight. Dieting seldom results in feeling happy with oneself; healthy eating and lifestyle habits, on the other hand, add to the pleasure of living. My patient Gail, 54, puts it this way: "There are things you can't change about your body ... but I think if you're feeling better your attitude tends to be better about your body too. It's all interrelated. You can't change your basic body build, but you feel so much better when you exercise, for example."

Resisting the Pressure To Be Thin

I'm not entirely clear as to how one can resist society's pressure to be unnaturally thin. For starters, one would have to confront or overlook on a daily basis comments about body size, most often in association with remarks about overeating, in books, movies and everyday conversation. Women are told to diet and not to gain weight and yet are tempted by "decadent" treats, which I guess people see as a reward for being so abstemious in their daytime eating. My best advice is to consult those books and websites (see Further Reading, p. 159) that promote a non-dieting, self-esteem building approach to life. Strive to feel as good about yourself as Glenda, 47, does: "I feel really good about me. I used to look in a mirror and I used to go, Oh God. Now I look in a mirror and it's like, Right on."

Or learn to accept your natural body size the way Linda, 38, does:

> If I was supposed to be tall and thin, I wouldn't be 5 foot 3 and a little bit round. This is my body, I'm happy with it. I think I'm fine. And if people comment on my food intake? So? I'm eating. I enjoy my food. I like food. If I didn't eat I would be 110 pounds and I would be sick and I wouldn't be able to do my job and look after my family. But I eat, not at regular hours, I eat when I get hungry and, too bad.

The comedienne Sandra Shamas addresses the subject of body acceptance. In a review of her 2002 stage show, *Wit's End, Heart's Desire*, she was quoted as saying, "I've been mad at my body for so long that I'd forgotten what the argument was about." She resolves her dilemma by quipping, "I don't know what my problem was; it was holding up my head just fine."

You will find a lengthier discussion of self-esteem at the end of this chapter, as we need high self-esteem to overcome all the barriers to healthy eating.

The Inability to Apply Knowledge to Ourselves

The third barrier to healthy eating that I've identified in my work with my patients is an inability to apply knowledge to ourselves. What I have discovered in my job at Health Watch is that the women I see do know their nutrition, but somehow they see their knowledge as applying to everyone else. "My children eat breakfast" or "I pack lunches for my children" are statements I often hear. My favourite comment on this theme came from a woman who raises show dogs. At one point in our conversation she said to me, "Do you mean I should be feeding myself the same way I feed my dogs?" A farmer told me he notices that when he feeds his chickens cod liver oil they have shinier feathers. Why is it we can see the association between health and good food in children and even animals, but can't see that the same holds true for us? The women who feed their children breakfast seem almost to believe that the act is in some way magic, that if the children are fed, then the caregiver will be well fed by proxy. "There's always yogurt, milk, cut up vegetables, fruit ... in the fridge for the children," they say. And more than once a woman has conceded to me, "Well I suppose I could make my own lunch at the same time as I make the children's." Just as in an airplane adults are told to put on oxygen masks before helping the children (to ensure that they'll be able to help them), mothers have to take care of their own food needs along with those of their children. As my patient

Lynn, 48, has come to recognize, "I can't take care of other people if I don't take care of myself first." I sometimes ask women to eat the way they would like their children to eat, to pretend there is another child in the house — themselves.

Some women focus on taking care of their husbands rather than themselves. Clara, 64, offers some excellent advice to them:

> I've been married for forty-five years and what I told my husband is that I cannot love anybody else unless I love myself first. And I firmly believe that. I think if you're not happy with your own personality, if you cannot say to yourself, okay I'll have to deal with this, he's not going to be here all the time so I have to sort of centre on myself, then I will have nothing else for him or anybody else.

Overcoming the Inability to Apply Knowledge to Ourselves

With regards to this habit many of my patients have of feeding their loved ones well but not themselves, the best I can do at Health Watch is to remind them that their health is equally important to that of their family members. They must look after themselves, I point out, in order for them to continue to look after their children and their partners. They also have an opportunity to act as wonderful role models for their children. Not only can they demonstrate healthy eating and activity habits, they can help their children develop the ability to consider their own welfare along with the welfare of others.

Building Self-Esteem

Our best intentions to regularly refuel our bodies, eat healthy foods and generally take good care of ourselves may well come to nothing if we do not pay attention to building our self-esteem. In fact, I believe self-esteem may be the core value that we need in order to look after ourselves. Women are generally encouraged from childhood on to be caregivers, and often put their own needs last. But in the long run this pattern is not sustainable — there must be some balance. In an article published in 1994 in *Wellness Management*, the newsletter of The National Wellness Association (Wisconsin), self-esteem is identified as the critical factor in change. "Wellness is caring enough about yourself to take stock of your life, make the necessary changes and find the support to maintain your motivation." Unfortunately, the needed support is not always readily visible. Women are expected to be caregivers, both of children and of ailing parents, regardless of what other work responsibilities they have. Women who work outside the home often feel tremendous pressure at their jobs. I believe that many women feel guilty about taking time or doing anything for themselves. I sometimes point out that they would probably give away a bonus five minutes that might appear in their day.

Popular culture is often unsupportive to women's self-esteem. I recently read about a survey that showed overweight women feel discouraged about ever achieving the ideal body weight portrayed in the media. In fact, their self-confidence is undermined by all the photos glamourizing super-thin women, and in response they follow unhealthy diet plans instead of focusing on healthy eating and exercise. This issue was recognized by Dr. C. Everett Koop, former Surgeon General of the United States, who once commented, "Preoccupation with body image is undermining and diverting energy that is better invested in healthful changes in behaviour."

Dietitians have contributed to this problem. One of my patients told me about once being forced to wear a paper pig on her forehead while in the waiting room of the clinic she was attending because she had not lost the requisite number of pounds. What a blow to her self-esteem that dietitian delivered! When I was an inpatient dietitian I twice was greeted with tears merely because I walked into the patient's room and introduced myself as the dietitian. Large women, in particular, often have a very long history of trying to lose weight and of being chastised for not succeeding by dietitian and doctor alike.

In such a climate, no wonder so many women lack the level of self-esteem needed to maintain healthy eating and exercise habits. It truly is a personal challenge to each of us to build the reserves of self-appreciation and love we need to overcome the many factors pressuring us to adopt unhealthy habits. We do know that people are more likely to improve their eating and exercise habits if they feel good about themselves. Many women who come to Health Watch have this kind of self-esteem, and their words eloquently demonstrate the kinds of attitudes that foster healthy choices. Mildred,

64, explains that in her view, "You are your own best friend."

Thea, 51, taught me about the importance of self-acceptance:

> You have to look at yourself from the outside
> and really be able to accept all the good in
> you. You also need to be able to look at your-
> self and say, Hmmm I'm not so terrific in
> these areas, but not get hung up about it.
> That knowledge is what's going to help you
> in all the little situations you're going to find
> in your life.

Recognizing that to help others you must take care of yourself is the point made by Sarah, 69: "I know that I'm going to do what's right for me. I have to consider myself first before I'm able to do something for other people."

Linda, 38, rightly reminds us that we all have the right to demand the same dignity and respect, regardless of our size: "You may be a size three on the outside and I may be a size thirteen on the outside. But inside we still are the same thing. You treat people how you want to be treated. You treat with respect and people will treat you with respect."

I would also like to share some tips for building self-esteem that are posted on the National Cattlemen's Beef Association Web site, entitled "Top 10 Everyday Solutions for the Everyday Hero." We have these tips on a bulletin board in our waiting room at Health Watch.

Top 10 Everyday Solutions for the Everyday Hero

1. Relish food. Food is a pleasure, not a foe. Rid yourself of strict diets and restrictive eating. Eating well — and eating enough — energizes every day.

2. Enjoy movement. Dance, stroll, stretch, garden — whatever you choose gives you a health boost.

3. Appreciate your beauty. Cast off negative attitudes about your body. Admire it, dress it, groom it and pamper it. Do it now, rather than later.

4. Trust yourself. Tune in to your inner signals. You'll discover when you've eaten enough, need a long walk or require more rest.

5. Savour some down time. It's all about you ... a nap, a massage, a good book or a bubble bath leave you relaxed, refreshed and ready for your responsibilities.

6. Decompress stress. When you feel over-whelmed, pause for some perspective. Close your eyes and take a few deep breaths. Even a small break helps restore calm and clarity.

7. Give up guilt. An unread report, a dusty house or a fast food meal for the kids doesn't make you a bad person.

8. Focus on your priorities. Say no to requests that overburden you. Protect and cherish time for your loved ones — and for yourself.

9. Ask for help. Don't try to be a superhero. Even Everyday Heroes don't have to do it all themselves. Family, friends and neighbours usually are glad to lend a hand — just as you do for them.

10. Remember you're #1! If you love yourself first, everything else will fall into place. To accomplish anything, you need to love yourself.

© Council for Women's Nutrition Solutions and National Cattlemen's Beef Association

I can think of no better way to help people than by identifying the barriers to healthy eating. Once people realize what these barriers are, it is up to them to decide to what extent they can overcome them. The task is not easy. As I've discussed here, many factors interfere with our self-esteem. I also often point out to my patients that life gets in the way of the pursuit of health, and many of my patients confirm this for me. They have found, as have I, that being adequately fuelled and nourished lowers the risk of getting sick and ultimately makes life easier and more enjoyable.

PART 2

FUELLING THE MIND AND SPIRIT

The Wise Women of Health Watch

Introduction

The chapters you've just read have given you an in-depth explanation of my views on nutrition — I've told you exactly what I tell my patients. Now it is time for me to talk about what I have learned from them and to let you know why I refer to them as the Wise Women of Health Watch.

My fascination with my patients started as soon as I arrived at the clinic. Every day I was invited into thoughtfulness, though I was not aware of the dynamic for quite a while. Over time I came to see that on a regular basis, the women I met with would naturally reveal something of themselves or their attitudes that would strike me as being important. As I became more attuned to the fact that this was happening, I realized that the statements I was hearing were relevant to reading I was doing at the time on the determinants of health. I was immersed in these principles at a wellness conference I attended shortly after beginning to work at Health Watch. For one week I attended lectures by dynamic and exciting "wellness leaders" who taught me that we need to look at the whole person, not just at bodily functions, to help a patient improve their overall health. I learned that people who are able to find enjoyment in the things they do and people who can connect to others and to their environment are the people who achieve health. People who do volunteer work, for example, are happier and healthier than those who don't. The lecturers' perspectives took into account not just body, but mind and spirit as well. My interest in my patients expanded. I started to ask questions that did not necessarily relate to the amount of calcium in their diets or how many vegetables they ate. Instead, I started to ask them what they thought about health in general and what brought them to Health Watch. Then I began asking about the ways in which they dealt with different aspects of their lives. I made recordings and took notes. I believe that I see a unique group of people at Health Watch, people who truly care about their health. Many of them already have their answers to my questions figured out.

The women I see never seem to mind my questions and very generously share their insights. I am hoping that eventually their thoughts will help me arrive at a satisfactory answer to the question of how one can influence someone else to adopt healthy behaviours. I'm looking for specific methods of inspiring healthy behaviour that I can pass on to those who may not be easily motivated, and so far I have only clues.

When I talk with patients who are obviously following a healthy lifestyle, I start off with the query, "Have you always done things this way?" Most often the answer is "Yes." These patients might cite a mother's or a father's example, early family behaviours, a natural liking of healthful food or a natural liking of physical activity as strong influences on their lifestyle. The wellness movement believes that self-esteem and realizing that we are responsible for our own health are important factors in providing the motivation to follow healthy life practices. Perhaps it is these factors in the Health Watch women that motivate them, rather than the natural liking for good food or exercise to which they attribute their motivation. They are naturally self-motivated. It may be that there is a limit to how much influence an outside person can have in motivating others. But I like to think that hearing about the lessons learned and positive experiences of others can help us when we are seeking support for making healthy changes.

In this next part of the book, I share my patients' wisdom. I see this part of the book as providing potential fuel for the mind, heart and spirit, in contrast to my opening chapters, which look at how to fuel the body. I hope that you will find much here that energizes your daily life. Numerous quotations from my conversations with my patients both guide and illustrate the discussion. As mentioned in the introduction, I have changed the names of the women quoted to preserve practitioner-patient confidentiality. The only woman whose name I did not change was very firm, the last time I talked to her, that she would like her real name used. Marg Brown, please enjoy this part of the book!

6

Fuelling Change:
The Factors that Motivate Healthy Choices

Not every woman puts staying healthy at the top of her priority list. What is it that makes some people conscientious about their health and others not? What makes some people cautious and others careless? As a health care professional, I very much want to understand what motivates people to work at staying healthy. I can't help but think that if we knew the answer to that question, we could put it to use helping people establish healthy lifestyles.

I thought I had made a great discovery one day at the clinic. We are continuously revising the patient questionnaires that patients answer at each visit. The questionnaire is meant to capture the particular complaints the patient may have as well as elicit certain information that guides discussion. For instance, in the diet section we ask for a sample day's menu, the number of meals typically eaten away from home, and the number of servings of dairy foods eaten daily. An earlier version of the form asked questions about immunizations, dentist visits and the wearing of seatbelts. As these questions were not relevant to the visit at hand, but were really meant to remind people to do these healthy things, they were later taken off the form. However, while those questions were on the form, I noticed a curious thing — people who seemed to show no interest at all in healthy habits, that is, people who didn't seem to care if they ever ate a vegetable (my own personal gasp inducer), didn't sleep enough hours, drank a lot of alcohol, smoked and so on, also did not wear seatbelts. Now if I run across a person with poor health habits (rare indeed at our clinic), I ask, seemingly out of the blue, "Do you wear a seatbelt?" The person is usually surprised by my question, but I am seldom surprised by the answer. What is the relationship between not wearing a seatbelt and not eating vegetables? I have come to believe that the people who exhibit this pattern truly do not see a relationship between present behaviour and future health. I have therefore come to feel that a certain amount of what I would call "healthy fear" may be important.

Diverse factors seem to motivate those patients who do eat their vegetables and wear seatbelts. Some women explain their healthy habits simply, saying, "I've always done things this way." Some come to them at particular stages of life — when they are pregnant, for example, when they reach menopause or when they first start to feel the aches and pains that come with ageing. Some change their habits because they want to be good role models for their children. Many women alter their way of eating when their husbands need a special diet, many more because they are concerned about their weight.

Most people have what I refer to as healthy fear when it comes to illness. Almost a mirror reflection of this fear is another very strong motivating factor for adopting habits to assure health: the love of life. Many of the women of Health Watch want to stay healthy because they want to live well and for a very long time.

In the rest of this chapter, I explore the most common themes that emerge as women explain to me what motivates them to make healthy choices.

Fear of Illness

The death or illness of a family member or friend often triggers reflection on their own health in my patients. Sometimes relatively young people develop an interest in health after seeing their parents hooked up to machines, stricken by heart disease or cancer. Jane, 60, believes that if "people go to a nursing home and see all the people there, stooped over, they would say, 'No, I don't want that.'" Annette, 45, stopped smoking because she didn't want her children to smoke and because, working in a hospital, she was in daily contact with people on respirators. She told herself that if she turned eighty-five or got a terminal illness, then she would give herself permission to start smoking again.

Sometimes the fear of illness hits even closer to home. Many people don't see a need to change behaviour when they feel good and are basically healthy. A diagnosis of high blood pressure or a blood test that returns high cholesterol readings acts to motivate a closer look at diet, exercise habits and the role of personal responsibility in maintaining well-being. As Sally, 54, put it after being told her choles-terol was high: "We have to be responsible for ourselves. You don't wait until you're sick and then run to see the doctor to help you."

Many women have a fear of getting breast cancer. My patients are no different. They come to Health Watch because they know they will get competent and thorough screening for this disease. Women who have seen relatives struck with this illness often have especially strong clarity about what motivates their healthy lifestyle choices:

> I eat the way I do because that's the control that I have in my life. Both my parents have had heart problems, my mom and my aunt had cancer and the only control I have is food and exercise. And so if I can take that control, myself, hopefully I'll remain healthy. Maybe not, but at least I'll have done everything I can do for myself. If you're eating healthy foods, hopefully you're mak-ing your body strong enough that you can resist anything.
>
> ROBERTA, 46

Ageing

At a certain point in life, people become aware that they are getting older. One of my Health Watch patients told me that she saw life as a hill that you climb, and all of a sudden, one day you are able to see what life holds for you on the "down" side of the hill. Health Watch patients want to live long and healthy lives despite the ageing process and that motivates them to take charge of their health. Karen, 45, exemplifies this attitude when she says: "When I was thirty-five I decided that I had to prepare myself for older life. I didn't want to end up like my grandmother, in a nursing home."

It's not only the desire to avoid illness and dependency that motivates my patients. They want to enjoy an active, pleasurable retirement:

> When I get older I don't want to be decrepit. I want to be active and enjoy life. I want to travel and hike and bike and all that. I don't want to just sit somewhere and not be able to do stuff because I'm overweight and my muscles are weak and I have osteoporosis.
>
> JILL, 45

Their commitment to health means that many of the women I counsel either break stereotypes or are preparing to do so. Jane, 48, says, "When I'm eighty I want to go to Hawaii and learn to surf." Her role model could be my seventy-year-old patient Serena who sails and who celebrated her last birthday by sky diving!

Jill, Jane and Serena are talking about having fun and continuing to look forward to having fun at every age. They demonstrate a commitment to achieving what the wellness movement declares we need to be healthy — the ability to play. Such people are likely to reach retirement in a healthy state.

Weight Concerns

Much as I try to fight the thinness movement, I must also acknowledge that the desire to lose weight is a strong motivator for change. Women often start to gain weight in the middle decades of life. In pursuit of a thinner profile, they finally start exercising and watching the quality of their diets. Some turn to weight loss programs such as Weight Watchers which provide goals, structure, motivation and routine, including the weekly weigh-in, that people find attractive. I find it endlessly fascinating and frustrating that women often will not give up unhealthy eating habits unless they are "on a diet." At the same time, I am glad that this desire motivates some women to adopt a healthier lifestyle:

> I changed my eating habits because I needed
> to lose weight but I wanted to do it health-
> ily so I wouldn't put all that weight back on
> again. I knew I had to change the way I ate.
> Health is very important to me now, more so
> because I'm diabetic and I know I have to
> look after myself because of that.
>
> GLENDA, 47

There remains a danger if the only goal of diet change is to lose weight. If the expected weight loss is not achieved, the motivation for continuing the healthy changes may diminish. Glenda, however, has decided to lose weight for the sake of her health, not because of social pressures.

Children's Health

We are role models for our children, and although some women preach and don't practise, others strive to set a good example. Many of the women I see, in fact, realize that their children often learn much more from watching their parents than from being told what to do. Roberta, 46, explains, "I have two girls and I feel that I'm their role model. If I don't eat in a healthy fashion, they're going to say, well I can have the cookies, too, or I can have the chips, too. They're watching, all the time."

For some women, the realization that they are a role model for their children helps them make the change to better habits:

> I started to eat healthy because I wanted my kids to eat that way. I had to change the way I was eating in order for them to follow me. I used to eat like whenever. Now I like to have a bowl of fruit on the counter and I buy salads in a bag so they can just open the fridge, grab a tomato out of the bowl and make a tomato sandwich. They always eat healthy. I feel good and my kids are never sick, ever. I tell people it's because they eat healthy.
>
> SHELLEY, 43

As I've stated in Part 1, Health Watch women make sure their children's diets are balanced even when they do not necessarily follow the same dietary standards for themselves. But the women who practice the "do what I do, not just what I say" philosophy can only benefit from the improved diet they will achieve by actually eating the same way they want their children to eat. And the children will most likely continue to eat in this healthy pattern when they reach adulthood. Women are also tremendously influenced by the needs of their partners.

Partners

Many women experience a strong impetus to change their behaviour when their life partner's health deteriorates. If a partner develops diabetes or heart disease, the whole family's diet and exercise habits frequently change to reflect the new recommended protocols. Sadly, a health crisis often kick-starts people into doing things in ways they had long planned, but somehow had never gotten around to before. They start walking and start watching the quality of their diets. When one partner has to follow a diabetes meal plan, the other often starts eating the same way. Elizabeth, 73, told me that it was her husband's death that motivated her to change and to pay more attention to her health: "Now I had to look after the house and the garden all by myself and I didn't want to get all crocked up."

Partners can also motivate unhealthy behaviour. Some of my patients do not serve vegetables at meals because their husbands will not eat them. I remind women to stay focused on what they believe is best for them, regardless of a partner's eating preferences.

Advice From Others

Despite the movement toward use of alternative health practices, people still rely on traditional medicine (hence their visits to Health Watch). I have found that advice from the doctor exerts a powerful influence on my patients — they don't necessarily do everything their doctor, or anyone else, recommends, but advice from her or him figures heavily in health decisions. For instance, I have counselled numerous women to take a calcium supplement if unable to consume enough calcium in their diets. However, it is only after I hear the words, "My doctor told me to take calcium pills," that the woman takes the suggested action. Sometimes helpful advice comes from a mother, a daughter, a sister, a neighbour. One of my favourite allies was an unexpected one. After years of hearing one woman tell me that she hated taking pills, she arrived one year and told me she was now taking a calcium supplement. The reason? She had heard Oprah explain that taking calcium keeps one young.

Many people feel uncomfortable wavering too far from the actions recommended by their doctor. I have had particular problems when recommending multivitamin supplements, as my patients frequently respond, "My doctor says that my diet is fine and I don't need them." I may disagree with the doctor, but I note how much influence that doctor has. The depth of the faith some people place in their doctors is very clear in a statement Rose made to me:

> If something happens and you have to go to
> the hospital, believe in the doctor who's
> telling you and do it. Don't try to figure you
> know better than someone else, because you

don't. That person's been trained in what
they're doing and they're only doing it to
help you. So every time they said to me you
need an operation, I had it. And every time
they said you needed this, I went ahead. I
don't feel that I know everything.

ROSE, 90

Not all Health Watch women listen so attentively to
their physicians. Nor do they so readily accept advice without giving it critical thought. They realize that their situations and their lives are unique and that any piece of advice
has to be measured against what they know to be true about
themselves. Health Watch women like to give and receive
advice but they are generally determined and very able to
make decisions for themselves. I, myself, am very fond of
advice. I like to hear others' opinions on topics that I am
thinking about. I particularly like it when I receive the same
advice from two separate sources — force in numbers,
perhaps.

Some women I meet are uninterested in following
advice on healthy habits and this confuses me. I often ask
them, "Why is it that you don't feel motivated to change?"
Their answer is usually quite simple: they do not see any
need to change. They feel good, they feel they have family
longevity on their side, and they don't desire to endure the
discomfort involved in changing their behaviour just for
some possible future benefit. One woman told me that she
is a fatalist. Her father died from lung cancer and she continues to smoke; when it's her time to go, she'll go. One

patient told me that she only felt unwell after she stopped smoking. Once she started again, she resumed her former feeling of wellness. And of course, there are no guarantees that we will live long, healthy lives by following all the health precepts put before us. Not getting your calcium, for instance, does not necessarily condemn you to osteoporosis. Eating a healthy diet is a leap of faith for some. In thinking about these issues, I'm reminded of a joke I once heard, about a man being shown around heaven. Everything was so wonderful, he finally turned to his wife in anger, saying, "If it hadn't been for your bran muffins, I would have been here ten years earlier."

Love of Life

Health Watch patients love living. They love their families and their friends, they love to travel, to garden, to golf. They love their jobs. Their strong love of life is evident in the energy they bring to their Health Watch visits — the sound of laughter in the waiting room often sets a wonderful tone in the clinic. My patients do not want to miss the challenges and pleasures of even one day and aim to live their lives to the fullest. As Margaret, 83, says, "I like my life. I live every day to the fullest." Mariah, 89, tells me, "I love every day." In fact, I often feel that the women who come to Health Watch experience each day as a gift and can barely wait to wake up each morning to see what the day holds for them. Their enthusiasm is contagious — it's hard, for instance, not to be swept up into Abigail's love of everything that touches her:

I love people and I love kids. That doesn't mean that I can't be upset with someone but I really like them. I like to be alone, too. I really like me best of all. I don't know if that's part of it or not. In order to be positive you have to like yourself. I love where I live. I had a wonderful career, too. I sort of look on old age as you get paid back. And it's been wonderful.

ABIGAIL, 64

Abigail has mentioned several factors that are important in living a healthy life, without having read a word by the wellness movement authors! She connects with other people, yet she takes time alone to connect with herself. She is conscious of the choices she makes and derives pleasure from her life. She has high self-esteem. All Health Watch women share all or some of these attitudes. Books have been written about the healing power of laughter and laughter is often the prevailing atmosphere in the Health Watch waiting room.

But are Health Watch women healthier because they love life or are they able to enjoy life more because they are healthy? I can't really answer this question. Certainly, staying healthy can only contribute to the ability to fully enjoy life. Leila, 57, keenly appreciates this fact when she says, "I don't want to ever feel like an old lady but I want to live to a ripe old age. And I want to get there healthy."

I've presented here what my patients tell me about why they do their best to make healthy choices in life. Now I'd like to examine one of the most important "hows" of keeping a healthy life on track — the cultivation of attitudes that fuel healthy living.

7

Attitudes That Fuel Healthy Living

Many of the women who come to Health Watch have developed certain attitudes that help them live their lives in good health. I am constantly struck by how these attitudes help them cope with life's difficulties. The women daily demonstrate to me that life is shaped by our attitudes to it, and as my patients say, to live a good life, you need a good attitude. In their book, *Healthy Pleasures*, Robert Ornstein and David Sobel write about how healthy people enjoy small, simple pleasures, and how they believe that things generally work out for the good. They demonstrate convincingly that healthy people are also absorbed in life and that their connectedness to others and to the world at large keeps them healthier than less connected people; they live longer too. Health Watch women demonstrate these healthy attitudes. They engage in life and have a great capacity for love.

There are eight key attitudes I explore here: attitudes towards taking control, ageing, life, stress, health, food, friends, and a partner's death.

Taking Control

The women who visit Health Watch sometimes come without their doctor's approval. They like the extra time they are given, the wider scope of services available than in the typical doctor's practice (including nutrition counselling and physiotherapy), and the fact that they see the written results of all their tests. These women want to be active partners in their health care. As Sharon, 52, says, "We are all in control of our own health and can't depend on anyone else to do it for us."

Taking control means seeking advice, exploring options and taking steps to change what can be changed. My patients ask many questions, often see both alternative and conventional medical practitioners and alter their diets or exercise regimes if they feel it would be helpful to do so. Each step of the way is taken thoughtfully and deliberately.

Many women I see elect to take control because they feel a strong responsibility to stay healthy — they do not want to become a financial burden on our public health care system:

> I try [to do] everything in moderation, eating, drinking, exercise, and I basically let my body tell me what I can and can't do. Of course I come for my yearly check-ups here [Health Watch] and I go for my dental every three months whether I want to or not and these things I feel are my preventive medicine back-ups ... Why should I be a burden

on the health system when it's so easy to do
these sensible things?

ESTHER, 70

Taking control can be life-saving as well. I have heard many stories of women's concerns being ignored by their health professional. Sometimes it is only after persistent demands that a breast lump that turns out to be cancerous is finally investigated.

My patients who take responsibility for their own health avoid affixing blame or looking backward; with them, the attitude that they are in charge of their own lives prevails:

I don't like to preach to people ... but I do try to point out, especially to other women, that we need to be looking after ourselves, that we need to take responsibility for it. It's very easy for women to blame things on somebody else or on this or that or the other thing. Well look at yourself and get a grip.

SALLY, 54

One thing you have to do is stop feeling sorry for yourself. You're responsible for your own life, no matter what your parents did to you or your husband did. You've got to go forward, and do it with a positive attitude. If you don't, you get stuck.

KAREN, 45

Given my experience here, I now take for granted that the women of Health Watch are, simply by their presence at the clinic, taking control. I believe that being in control makes people more secure and therefore stronger and more able to deal with whatever health challenge may come their way.

Ageing

Some of the women who visit Health Watch have been doing so for decades and many more have been patients for the past several years. "Just how long have I been coming?" is a question I'm often asked. As I look back through the reports to find the date of the woman's first visit, I'll occasionally find the record of a life threatening condition discovered on a yearly visit; many give credit to Health Watch for the early detection and intervention that has allowed them to reach their senior years. Through good health and illness, the women of Health Watch have aged with the clinic; how they view their ageing is key to their ability to stay healthy. Indeed, their example has been instrumental in shifting my own attitude to growing older! Consider Lorraine's sensible outlook:

> I like getting older. Not only do we not have
> any control over it, but I think the secret is
> to enjoy whatever age you are at and what
> comes with that age because once the whole
> thing unfolds, different things happen as we
> get older. So, just enjoy life. You have no

control over how fast it's going to go or how
slow it's going to go.

LORRAINE, 65

The women of Health Watch like the wisdom that ageing brings. As Julia, 66, explains, "Certainly I'm much
smarter and wiser than I was twenty, thirty, forty years ago,
oh yes." Stephanie echoes another common theme, the
greater inner freedom that comes with the years:

Getting older means more confidence, more
comfort in what you do and how you do it.
It's like you grow into yourself. I can do that
now because I'm old enough. I think you go
through a stage in your life where you feel
you have to please people. You get to a point
in your life where you are confident enough
that you can say, I need this, and you're comfortable doing that. You need it for yourself.
You have to know what you need and not
have the guilt associated with putting yourself first. And I think once you start to feel
that way and do that, others have a greater
respect for that.

STEPHANIE, 49

Some see old age as a state of grace, a very special phase in
life:

I have a few older women in my life and

those that I admire are the ones who haven't fought age. They accept themselves. They're not competing against younger women. I feel that I had my time as a younger woman. You have to leave space for the next people coming up. You reach the age of grace, that time when you have acceptance of yourself, with what you've done, what you didn't do, your disappointments, your priorities. There are certain things you didn't do. So you can look back at that and say, well I didn't do that but my energy level or my circumstance didn't allow for everything, so what I picked I succeeded in. Put that aside and move forward to grace, a new era of acceptance, of new opportunities and in a sense, spirituality.

ADAH, 60

I've tried to elicit from my patients secrets of healthy ageing, and so far I haven't discovered any magic formula. Most healthy older women think that's just the way they are. One advised me that a good face cream made all the difference to how you look as you age. Another seventy-five-year-old woman responded to my direct questions with, "You want to know the secret to a healthy life? Get down on your knees and scrub the kitchen floor."

While they're willing to talk about ageing with me, not many women I see feel old. I often ask my patients, "How old do you feel?" Their answers are not surprising to me, since I don't feel any older myself than I did even twenty years ago. The seventy-five-year-old floor scrubber I describe above told me that she felt she was seventeen. She went on to explain that although she doesn't feel old, she does recognize that it takes her a bit longer to recover after an energy expenditure. Esther, 70, provides another example of this spirited approach to life: "Forget about your age. If you're fit, you carry on and you just think of yourself as a young person and you do all the things that you did as a young person. I think I'm in my thirties."

Indeed, the women of Health Watch emphatically do not believe that old age has to be about a sagging body and ill health. Rather, like Freda, 73, they focus on the continuing growth and learning life offers: "When you reach sixty you realize how little you know. There's so much to learn."

They find age brings with it a new capacity for acceptance and forgiveness:

> As you get older you become aware that we're human and making mistakes is not a major event. It's just part of life, it's not a big deal. As you get older, you realize what's important and it's smelling the roses, walking in the woods, and having your children, being able to hug them and support them and smile.
>
> SHERYL, 61

They are inspired by what lies ahead:

I have a mother ninety-nine years of age and she's in her own home, takes care of herself, has a garden. And she has a steady stream of younger people coming to visit her and she really acts like a counsellor to them. They think they're doing her a favour by coming to visit when in fact I think it's the other way around. I have watched her evolve from sixty to ninety-nine and what a range of change there has been in her attitudes and so on. I would certainly say she's an extraordinarily wise woman at this point. Maybe you just have to live long enough.

HILDA, 62

As I've already mentioned, my own attitude to ageing has been strongly affected by the women who come to Health Watch. Instead of fearing getting older, I now see it as a way of getting smarter and more in tune with myself. Every day I see wise, vibrant women of all ages struggling with the different things we all deal with in life, but taking from life all it has to give. One of my own personal goals in life is to become more mellow. Wasn't I blessed one day by a woman who related her own story to me? When I asked her about a particular situation and how she handled it, she said, "Well, you know, when you get to be seventy, you get kind of mellow." I have a lot to look forward to.

Life

The women at Health Watch have endured their share of illness and loss. They also deal daily with tough tasks like raising a family, working at a difficult job, battling depression. Many stop, when relating their present philosophies or happiness, to remind me that they have dealt with hardships in their lives. They are telling me that life is not always easy, but with the right approach, it can still be a positive experience. Janet, 63, adopted the sailor's saying, "You can't change the winds but you can adjust your sails" as a keystone of her approach to life. She translated this adage as, "You cannot always help what has happened to you but you certainly have a choice as to how you deal with it." Her outlook is typical of the attitudes my patients bring to their life challenges. Eleanor, for instance, admires her mother for not letting an accident bring her down:

> My mother will be 92 the first of May this year and she fell and broke her nose and both wrists and when anybody would ask her how she is she'd say, "Oh I'm doing pretty good, you know, it could have been a lot worse; I could have broken my hip, and been in the hospital."
>
> ELEANOR, 68

Eleanor's mother sounds to me a lot like my patient Mary, 51, who says, "I have a friend who has a cup that is always half-empty, and I believe that mine is always half-full." Sometimes we see our blessings when we realize that others have not been so fortunate. The following story illustrates this:

> My husband had a severe health problem.
> He had to go and have open heart surgery at
> age twenty-four ... after I waited eight hours
> ... the surgeon finally came out and said to
> me, "Your husband will be fine." And right
> beside me sitting in the waiting room was a
> young lady who was twenty-one and her
> husband had a brain aneurism and the surgeon came out and took her aside and she
> started to cry. I quickly realized that her
> husband had not survived surgery. I realized
> that day that I was very fortunate and that I
> would recognize that and go through with a
> positive attitude most days.
>
> KAREN, 45

I've also learned from the women of Health Watch that the attitude we bring to our past has a huge influence on how well we handle the present. An idea that has made a deep impression on me, and that I repeat to patients, is the one expressed by Mildred. Look back only to see how far you've come, she says; never berate yourself for not doing more:

> I always try to be encouraging and when
> people get down and depressed I always stop
> and say, well look over your shoulder and see
> how far you've come and congratulate your-

self. You have to have perspective on your life and not just look at the problems that you're surrounded with. You have to look at how much you've learned, how much you've grown, what a better person you are, what you've achieved since way back then and then you can look ahead and see the promise of the future.

MILDRED, 64

Mildred knows that the attitudes she expresses here are important for her health. She is not only compassionate towards others, she is kind and forgiving towards herself. It takes some people years of meditation or counselling to reach the place Mildred has.

Mena, age 60, has taught me that we have just as much ability to respond to our present circumstances as to our past in a health-supportive way. I wonder how many of us forget that we can often choose our moods? Mena says: "When I get up in the morning I have two choices: I can have a good day or I can have a bad day. I choose to have a good day."

Marg Brown is another of those people who choose to be happy:

This is Marg, happy person. In life you have to enjoy things as they happen, the small things, like that good latte, that good cup of coffee, meeting somebody, a phone call, just enjoying a sunset, anything like that. And I think you have to be a little like Oprah says, look for your spirit and what's inside you. And to me, if you don't enjoy the moment, you're only going to enjoy the occasion you have once a year when you're a happy person and the other fifty weeks out of the year you're going to be looking around for just the basics that are boring and repetitive. So, enjoy the moment. Catch a little sunlight every hour of the day. That's it. Bye. Marg

Dinah, 67, sums it all up when she says, "We only pass through this life once. So why not be happy? Things can't always run your way."

Stress

High stress levels seem to be a constant companion of today's lifestyles. It is during periods of extreme stress that women find it so hard to exercise, eat well and find time for relaxation and rejuvenation. But even as stress interferes with one's ability to take care of one's health, it creates increased requirements for nutrients and rest. The women at Health Watch have their share of stressful situations to deal with and have developed certain attitudes that help them cope. They learn to be realistic about what they can do, an attitude exemplified by Esther, 70: "You can only do so much. You do the very best you can, whatever it is, and after that, you can't worry about it." They recognize that they have some control over how they view situations. Gabrielle, 65, is careful to avoid what she describes as "harmful" negative thinking: "You catch yourself thinking a negative thought or trying to work out something for too long, then you just say to yourself, that's it. Sing a song, put a piece of music on or something that changes your mood."

The women of Health Watch recognize that the thinking patterns and typical moods of the people around them can affect their ability to cope. Women at Health Watch want to be with positive people like themselves:

> I've learned not to say, "How are you today?"
> with certain people because you get three
> hours of "Ooh." I just stay around happy
> people, people who are energetic. If they
> have a down day they'll say to me, "Give me
> a kick." And if I have a down day they'll say,
> "Smarten up, we've got this, this and this to
> do." You feed off who you hang around with.
>
> LILA, 42

Edith, 67, has a refreshing, guilt-free bluntness about her choice to avoid certain people: "I cannot waste my time being around negative people because they bring me down. I don't want to be brought down. Life is too short."

Stress brings out the need for many different coping mechanisms and strong personality traits. My patients have taught me that with age comes experience in coping with stress and acceptance of what can't be changed, and that by taking control of our thinking patterns we can alter how we view stress. Or we can ally ourselves with other positive people who will help us maintain a half-full cup attitude.

Positive people have a good sense of humour, and as already mentioned, humour has a documented health benefit record. Nina's story makes it clear how important laughter and light-heartedness are for keeping the harmful effects of stress away:

> I don't take things too seriously; you can't do that. I try to tell my husband not to take things too seriously. He takes it on too hard sometimes and that's why his blood pressure goes up so easily. He needs me for his laughter and things like that.
>
> NINA, 59

Charlene, 58, captured all of these coping skills when she completed her health form. In answer to the question about how she handles stress, she answered: "Pray and go to church, sleep, talk to a friend, listen to music, exercise and watch a funny movie."

Health

Most of the people who come to Health Watch have a great respect for their health. As Heather, 56, reminds us, "If you don't have your health you have nothing."

The women realize that how they look after themselves today does make a difference to their future well-being:

> It's sad when people don't care about their health. I want to live for a very long time, healthily. I don't want to be miserable. I want to be like the neighbour down the street who is out walking his dog. I want to

be eighty without the joint pain and the satisfactory state of mind where you can walk
happily at eighty years of age.

RACHEL, 28

People don't always manage to keep all their healthy habits going. I usually say, "Life gets in the way." But what is consistent in healthy people, I find, is the desire and the willingness to be healthy. We can only do what we can do. And since there is no such thing as being perfect, and because there are so many elements that go into the health equation, I firmly believe that what a person actually accomplishes sometimes becomes more important than what they are not yet able to do. Women are reluctant to acknowledge their accomplishments. They downplay what it is they do as not being important because they are looking ahead to the next challenge. I like to point out to these women just how many healthy things they already do, whether it involves nutrition, exercise or maintaining positive attitudes. I think that recognizing our accomplishments gives us motivation to continue with our present positive health practices and sets us up to meet the next challenge when we are ready. I remember Mildred's attitude of looking back at what you have accomplished rather than dwelling on what you have not done.

Health also has its intangible aspects. It was at the wellness conference that I first learned about the concept of getting away from strict numbers and measurements when considering health matters. "Who measures the serum fun level?" was an important question posed there that emphasized for me that there is more to health than what is shown by the numbers on a height and weight chart or the results of a lab test. Of course, these measurements are important, but they must be put into context. I regularly talk to patients who have diabetes and high blood pressure. Do I recommend dietary changes that will help them lower their risk of future health problems? Of course. But I will also look to see if the person knows how to laugh, help others and embodies the other qualities that we know to be associated with long life. I may refer them to a book by Robert Ornstein and David Sobel (which I have already mentioned), *Healthy Pleasures*. This book discusses the many ways that we bring health to our lives.

Paradoxically, sometimes the desire to be healthy can interfere with the light-heartedness and self-respect so important to good health. One woman who comes to Health Watch is particularly attentive to health advice she has been given or that she reads. One year, as we reviewed her diet, she admitted that she had been trying to drink one glass of wine every day, as she had read that this would decrease her risk of getting heart disease. The problem was that she did not like wine and the drinking of it was a burden for her. She was trying so hard to be healthy that she was doing something that she believed was right, even though it was not something she enjoyed. She was very relieved when I told her that she didn't really need to drink wine and could derive the same health benefits from modifying her diet in other ways. In her case, the quality I call "healthy fear" had grown to too large proportions.

Food

My patients' attitudes to health and to food are intertwined.
Health Watch patients know that food is important to their
health. Some recognize that what they eat has an immediate
effect on how they feel. Most believe that how they eat
influences their future health and that by eating well they
can reduce their risk of getting common illnesses, like heart
disease. Rachel sums up a healthy attitude to food well:

> When I eat the foods that I know are
> healthy, and I know that are good for me as
> well, from education and reading, just tast-
> ing and feeling the results makes me feel fan-
> tastic. It's not bulky, it's satisfying, yet it's not
> going to make me feel sick. It feels good. I'm
> totally in tune with my body.
>
> RACHEL, 28

Rachel is referring to a healthy eating pattern that is rea-
sonably easy to attain. She is not caught up in the preoccupation with individual foods or complicated patterns of
eating to which some people subscribe. It's a wonder that
we're not all terribly confused by the information overload
around food. I sometimes advise my patients to stop listening or at least to use their own judgement. Carried to an
extreme, a preoccupation with food can lead to orthorexia
nervosa, a condition defined and explained by Steven
Bratman in his book, *Health Food Junkies*. Orthorexics are
people who exhibit an obsessive preoccupation with the
quality of their diet (as opposed to people with anorexia

nervosa, who focus on the quantity of food eaten). The problem is not the nature of the diet itself, but the attitude toward it and the loss of sense of proportion. There are many ways to be a healthy eater but the quest for the perfect diet, or the perfect weight loss diet, for that matter, may be a roadblock on the road to health.

Friends

Many Health Watch patients come for their appointments in groups. Sometimes they are all members from one family. One such family group spans four generations (the fourth generation representative being in diapers but brought along for the ride). Group members may come from the same town or be friends who live in different areas but meet up at the clinic once a year. Often our waiting room is very lively, with much talking and laughing going on and the wonderful energy of people connecting with people filling the air. No doubt about it, my patients value their friendships. In my conversations with them, they repeatedly tell me how they receive support from their friends and find it important to give support as well.

Florence, 75, feels that her friends help her cope with difficulties: "I deal with stressful situations by talking to friends. I think friends and being with them are important. Don't isolate yourself in the house." Gabrielle, 65, appreciates her young friends: "I have so many young friends. I think you have to — to stay young."

Friends can help us stay safe:

> I have a buddy system. Every day I phone a
> girl I went to school with. I phone another

very good friend of mine who was with me through all the hard times when my husband was sick and I phone another friend I've known for fifty years every day. We don't talk for very long, just say, "Hi how are you doing?," just checking in. And if I don't, well then they know I'm either away or there's a problem. I figure that at my age anything could happen at any time so that hopefully if I don't answer the phone they'll check in to see why. It makes good sense doesn't it?

IMELDA, 77

Health Watch women nurture their husbands, parents, children and each other. They recognize that they receive many benefits from having friends, and are happy to give back to them. Mildred demonstrates just how forgiving and understanding it is possible to be:

I have a lot of friends who come to me because I am a good listener. They tell me all sorts of intimate things and bring me problems. I tell them I don't have any answers but I've lived a long time and I have a lot of questions that they might take to themselves and consider and that may be the start of them solving, isolating, figuring out what some of their problems are. Whatever it is, whatever your problems are, they fill up your whole screen, no matter how big or small they are. Just a few days after my husband died, one of my closest friends called and said, "How are you making out today?" and I had a terrible time because of a lot of other things that were going on as well, trying to cope with the reality of my life, and I just said, "Oh, thanks for calling, I'm the better for talking to you." Then she said, "Well I'm glad someone's all right, I went to this bad manicurist yesterday and she bummed up my nail and I'm going to have to go all the way back there today and have her put on this blinkin' nail polish." I started to laugh because if I didn't I would have cried. You see that was filling up her whole screen. It was the only thing that was really aggravating her and that she had to deal with that day. She didn't have to deal with the things that I was dealing with. And she was coming to me with them. She was coming to me with her little problem and I said, "Don't worry honey, you'll be okay."

MILDRED, 64

Stephanie told me a story that sums up very well the crucial, and sometimes money-saving, role friends can play for us:

> I also think that talking to other people is a form of self-therapy because you generally figure things out yourself as you talk. Probably the worst thing anybody can do is to tell you what they think you should do. What you should do is sit down and talk about it and you figure it out yourself as you're going. There was a period where I thought I should take some counselling. I went to two sessions and I sat there and I talked and she shook her head and agreed with everything I said. I paid $100 each time and I thought, what the hell am I doing this for? First of all, I'm figuring it out myself as I talk and secondly she's agreeing with everything I say and I think I probably know as much as she does. So I took a girlfriend out for lunch and I never went back.
>
> STEPHANIE, 49

Of course, many of our patients do seek professional help and have benefited from it. The Health Watch nurse takes on the role of directing women to appropriate counselling agencies.

In the high value my patients place on strong friendships I find that once again their everyday wisdom matches the teachings of the wellness movement. Social support and human connections are tremendously important in keeping us healthy.

A Life Partner's Death

The women I see devote a lot of energy to their partners. Some of my patients have had unhappy marriages or relationships but many have shared their lives with close and good friends and the loss of a partner leads to a particularly hard time in their lives. Some have shared with me how it was they were able to go on living after the death of a life partner. Joanne, 65, says, "I consider it as another chapter in my life."

Sarah describes very well how numbing the loss of her husband was and how her first concern was for her family members, for whom she had to show a brave face. What is interesting to me is how she needed time to come to terms with her loss, but that eventually her mourning had to give way, freeing her emotions and allowing her to help her family feel at peace.

> When I lost my husband my concern was for his mother whom I loved dearly. My concern was play a game so that they think you're okay. My family's big concern was how I was going to handle Christmas and I did. It was the following Christmas that was bad for me because then I could let my hair

down, so to speak. But it took a year. Literally I can remember walking down my street and finally realizing that the grass was green and the sky was blue. I had lost it. I had felt that I was encased in ice. And it helped me control my emotions and helped me get through it and helped other people believe that I was okay. I did realize there had to come a time for me. But I had to wait, I had to be sure that our families were at peace with that I was okay and then I had my time.

SARAH, 69

Imelda overcame her sense of grief and loneliness by embracing life:

My husband died seven and a half years ago ... you eventually realize ... life goes on ... I thought, well this is going to be a disaster, because how do you make a life at seventy? You only have two alternatives: you can either make a life or you can sit at home and vegetate. I don't want to do that. So I started phoning my friends. I was quite lucky to have quite a lot of really nice friends and whenever anybody said to me, would you like to do whatever it was, whether I wanted to or not, I said, I'd love to, and I started to go out ... pretty soon I was surprised to see that I had a life ... But you know what came as quite a surprise to me was the fact that I wasn't lonely and I didn't mind being alone ... but learning to live alone was difficult in that I was surprised in the fact that I had been doing things for him, not for myself. And once he was gone I couldn't be bothered doing it for myself. So, principally the big thing was food. You know, you survive on sandwiches, a cup of tea or something like that and gradually, it's taken about seven years, but gradually you discover you're hungry and you start to prepare a proper meal.

IMELDA, 77

Both of these women suffered terrible losses. But they show us that the will to live and the will to live well reasserts itself, even in times of sorrow.

As you can see, the attitudes that fuel my patients' healthy lives are not mysterious or unachievable. Still, the simplest things in life are often the hardest to take in, and I feel I have learned a great deal from my patients about how important it is to be positive, to take charge of your own life, and to embrace getting older for the wisdom it brings. In my patients' lives I see just how powerful these concepts are in a way that brings home to me that the health sciences still have much to learn from everyday people.

8

More Fuel for Healthy Living:
Advice

My job at Health Watch is to give advice, advice about nutrition. Health Watch women are happy to advise me in turn. One woman phoned me back the day after our meeting to complete her story with a piece of advice she considered critical for bringing our talk to a conclusion. It is of course each person's prerogative to decide if she wants to follow another's advice. I myself am always happy to at least listen to advice, even if I don't always choose to take it, perhaps because I'm growing older and more mature. I have here organized advice I've received from my Health Watch patients — you'll find general advice and advice about eating well, keeping active and managing family life.

General Advice
The advice that I have been given can be very simple. I have been told not to worry about next week: "Take each day as

it comes," says Polly, 64. I have been reminded by Dorothy, 76, that instead of getting mad at something, "Get it out of your system." Betty, 70, advises: "Never go to bed worried. What's behind you, you can't do anything about it. You can fix it tomorrow." Florence describes very well how to stay unruffled:

> If there's something wrong and you can do something about it, do it. If there's nothing you can do about it put it in the back of your mind and maybe later on you can do something about it, but for the time being don't clog up your mind with stuff that you can't do anything about. Be calm in your attitude to everything.
>
> FLORENCE, 75

Florence may well have given one of the lectures at the wellness conference. She follows some of the key rules for dealing well with stress: she thinks things through, tackles one thing at a time, does it calmly and knows how to live with the things she cannot change.

Mildred doesn't so much give advice here as relate the keystones of her approach to life:

> If my children remember me for anything I think three things come to the fore: the first one is love and close to that is laughter and the third is getting some joy in eating and eating properly, using healthy food that comes from the ground, that is part of life.

Sharing natural things and caring and good
fellowship, that's important to me.
MILDRED, 65

Sara, 49, wanted to have her voice heard as well as contribute to the advice section of my book. "Ice cream is good for your skin," she told me. "Put that in your book!" Sara was pointing out that pleasure is good for us and her words serve as a reminder about the importance of allowing ourselves enjoyment.

Eating Well Despite Life's Difficulties

The daily reality of living a life can make food preparation and meal eating challenging — life gets in the way of healthy eating! In particular, jobs get in the way. I have talked to many women who work through their lunch hours, some because they get caught up in the work, and some because they can't leave their work station. I got very excited one day encouraging one patient to talk to her boss and tell her that lunch is important. After all, I explained, a tired and hungry person cannot perform as efficiently as a rested and nourished one. "I am the boss," she replied.

Not only do most women work outside the home while the children are growing up, the children of today are very busy with after-school activities. Many people travel great distances to their place of work. With all the driving and juggling of different schedules such a lifestyle entails, there just is not much time left in the day to fit in healthy habits. In fact, after a lunch hour talk I gave on "Eating on the Run," two women approached me with their story. They worked full time and commuted to work. They had small children. "Do the best you can," I said. "Yours is a superhuman task." One patient who eats exceptionally well told me, "I was only able to do this when I retired." Still I am amazed at the number of women who make health a priority. They go for a run or walk after a tiring day at work and they carefully plan their food shopping and preparation in order to make healthy eating a possibility:

> I plan ahead. We eat very simple prepared food. When we buy fruits and vegetables, we buy enough for the week and we wash it all and we store it, in baskets or in containers with paper towels to absorb the moisture, so when we come home and I'm preparing Caesar salad I don't have to start and wash all that romaine lettuce. If I'm doing a stir fry it's all clean. That's one way that keeps us eating simply and in a healthy way.
>
> BEVERLEY, 55

I had a wonderful discussion with Glenda one day, a woman who takes all of her day's food to work. As I've already indicated, I encourage my patients to carry food with them on a daily basis. I ask them to take their breakfast to work if they have no time to eat it at home in the morning and I ask them to carry lunch. If a woman can't make her own lunch, I ask her to pack the vegetables and fruits that will probably be missing from a lunch that she buys. Glenda packs all three meals for a twelve-hour shift. What a role model for us all she is!

140

When I work my twelve-hour shifts I take my breakfast, my dinner, and my supper with me. And I prepare that the night before so it's sitting in my fridge when I get up in the morning. I've got to be at work at 6:00 in the morning. At about 8:00, I have my breakfast, then it's anywhere between 11:30 and 12:30 when I have my lunch; my supper break is usually at about 5:30 at night. In between I have my three snacks. My last snack is usually between 8:00 and 9:00 at night. I go for my walk when I get home at 7:00 or I take my hour break and go for my walk at work. I'll see the people around me eating fast food. That doesn't even interest me.

GLENDA, 47

What did Glenda and I go on to talk about? We compared notes on the type of bag she packs her food in and all its different sections, so well designed for good storage of solid, liquid, hot and cold foods.

I'll give Katie, 40, the last word on how to eat healthily despite everything: "It just becomes a habit. Instead of reaching for the junk food you reach for the healthy food. How to fit it all in? Health should come first; make it a priority."

Activity

Health Watch women are well aware of the health benefits of exercise. Some of them are naturally active and always have been — it seems easy for them to participate in physical activities. The favoured activity is walking. Some of the women I see complain about having to give up their morning walk because they had to get up so early to arrive for their Health Watch appointment on time! I am surprised by how many Health Watch women are golfers. Not being a golfer myself, I asked one woman, "What exactly is it about golf that is so addictive?" "That one good shot," she replied.

For those who may not be inclined to exercise, Beverley, 55, offers a perhaps surprising motivation. While she acknowledges that exercise is good for her body, she also points out that "It makes me strong in my spirit." For those who feel they lack time, Katie, 40, says, "Instead of watching TV at night, I go to the gym."

Annette knows that it is difficult to lose weight without exercise, and offers a solution for those who feel they lack the space needed for activity:

> When I had to lose that weight I exercised an hour and a half faithfully [every day] for at least two years. I also bought a cheaper version of the Stair Master and you don't need to follow a set pattern. I just do it when I watch television and I just step up, step down, step up, step down, step sideways, swing my arms. You need such little space.

It's unbelievable. Don't let people say that they can't exercise because they don't have the space.

ANNETTE, 58

If you still can't find a way to get active, note that even housework can contribute to your health through the physical effort you put into it. Leila could afford to have a cleaning lady but chose not to:

I will never have a cleaning lady. My husband hired a cleaning lady years ago and I fired her. I said, "Why is she getting healthier than me? She's running up and down the stairs and I'm sitting here reading a book, while she's getting healthy, doing my dirty work."

LEILA, 57

Managing Family Life

Every mother I've talked with confirms that it becomes more difficult to eat healthy food and exercise when there are young children to look after — available time simply shrinks. Even when women do not work outside the home, they still have to manage housework, make meals and take charge of transporting children to and from after-school activities — that's the reality of today's lifestyle.

When I hear my patients' stories I sometimes feel overwhelmed by the numbers of tasks people juggle on a daily basis. I understand that their children's needs come first and

I struggle to think of ways that they can introduce healthy habits into an already packed day. And I find it interesting to hear how successfully some people do manage their busy lives.

The key factor in managing family life, according to my patients, is being organized. Lorraine explains how she kept her family and herself organized and eating well after her marriage break-up:

> First of all you tell your kids the truth. You sit down and you say, listen, your dad isn't here anymore. It's you and me, that's it. We have a certain amount of time and ... money and we have to co-operate. If we don't co-operate or if you upset me, I'll be upset at work and I might lose my job ... And they understood that ... they knew the rules. They had their to-do lists on the fridge, the daily, the weekly and the monthly. And they knew that if we were going to live as a good family and enjoy everything that we could, we had to each do our own and share our own things. At supper the phone was taken off the hook. That was our family time together and we talked about things of the day and what went wrong or what was good.
>
> LORRAINE, 58

Barbara, 46, uses structure as her tool as well, explaining, "It's a matter of delegating tasks and being organized."

Health Watch patients number many grandparents among them. Some tell me how much they enjoy their grandchildren in a way they were not able to do when their own children were young and they were too busy. One woman told me a wonderful story about playing Harriet the Spy with her granddaughter. It's not strictly a story about managing family life, but it is a story about creating lasting good memories for our children. I'd like to end this section with this little tale about the magic of living well together. Isn't that what keeps us going, after all?

> So Grandma was Nancy Drew and she was Harriet the Spy and we went on a hunt in the mall to see who looked suspicious. She had her little magnifying glass and a little piece of paper to write down descriptions of shady characters. In the restaurant one chap she had been a little leery of got up to go to the washroom, so she took her magnifying glass over and carefully looked at his cup. It's a wonder we weren't charged with stalking! It was fun and she had a great time. And we were creating memories. You can impart some of the wisdom of life, some of the mistakes you've made, the fun things you've done, and somehow give that to the children, because they're the next generation, they can only benefit.
>
> SHERYL, 61

9

Common Threads

In my conversations with my patients, certain themes repeat themselves. From my perspective, these themes represent attitudes that are critical to being healthy because these attitudes provide the "core fuel" that energizes other healthy patterns of living. Most of the women of Health Watch enjoy life, feel a sense of gratitude for what they have, keep a positive outlook and have a strong sense of themselves. I call these attitudes "common threads" because I hear about them so often and because I feel both learning about them and living them weaves a pattern of pleasure and enjoyment in which I find myself happily getting caught. Health Watch women are people who have learned how to successfully find the good in whatever life has to give them.

Enjoying Life

Health Watch patients enjoy life. I can't even begin to count how many times I have been told this. It is this taking of pleasure in the everyday that motivates my patients to look after themselves — they want to live as long as possible and squeeze out the juice from every last bit of life given to them. They don't want to be sick and they don't want their lives to end. Every day brings pleasure. As Sybil, 69, says, "It's a blessing when you wake up in the morning." My patients also have a very strong sense of how to cultivate their enjoyment of life. Sybil points out that there is great pleasure to be found in helping others:

> You've got to enjoy what you're doing ... I always think that you should just get off your butt and get involved in something. I work in a hospital with kids and I love it. You know, you're doing something. You're contributing something. You have to do that. And you get back what you give, don't you?
>
> SYBIL, 69

Janie, 54, on the other hand, treasures her alone time, saying of her morning walk, "It's peaceful, it's quiet and if anyone wants to walk with me I feel I don't want them to. It's my time."

Rose relies on her sense of humour to keep life sweet:

> I can make fun of myself and of anybody. And I do think you need laughter because a real good laugh, what we used to call a belly laugh, will relax your stress so much more than any pills or anything else. Enjoy yourself. I have a very good life ... I believe in life

after death. I don't know what kind of life.
But if you look at flowers that die and ...
there's nothing there and next spring there's
a green sprout and there's your flower. And I
really believe that if there's a reincarnation of
a flower or a weed, why not of a human?

ROSE, 90

Thankfulness

The women who come to Health Watch have, in comparison to many people, exceptional health, and exceptional
physical capability to keep doing what they're doing. Yet
they do not take their health for granted — instead they
tend to be aware of and grateful for their good fortune. A
sentiment that I hear often from my patients is how lucky
they are in comparison to other people. Lorraine, 74,
considers herself to be "a lucky girl." Marianne, 56, enjoys
every day because she is "a very fortunate girl." The advice
my patients remember from a parent, or the advice they give
to their children, generally includes encouragement to see
how happy one's own situation looks in comparison with
others' misfortunes.

Even though Gabrielle, 65, has reservations about
getting older, she still chooses to focus mainly on how much
she has to be thankful for in her life: "I hate this ageing but
I'm so grateful that I have the lifestyle I have. My health is
good. I'm lucky that I was born in the right year and that I
had wonderful loving parents."

I believe that thankfulness is linked to spirituality. People with strong beliefs in a higher power or who have powerful connections with the earth and nature have been shown to be healthier people.

Positive Outlook

Being healthy allows one to be more positive. Or is it that being positive brings good health? Research indicates that having a positive attitude, indeed even believing that you are in good health, can lead to a longer life. I do believe that life is more enjoyable if you can focus on the good. My patients have learned to do that, to surround themselves with like-minded friends and to pass these attitudes on to their children. They consciously look for the positive in life. Sometimes when I ask the women who see me why they're positive and how they learned to be positive, I'm told, "I was just born that way." Other women, as the quotes in this section show, believe that a positive attitude is something we can learn to nurture. Whatever their explanation for their outlook, these women carry their positive attitudes into my office, and as a result, I am left feeling good. How much they must contribute to their family and friends!

How to maintain a positive outlook, then? Florence, 75, points out that we often have a choice about how we feel: "Remember the good things and forget the bad things. The choice is yours. Be positive about things. You have two choices, you may as well choose the best one, that's the way I look at it anyway."

Abigail, 64, notes that: "It's easy to be positive when you're healthy." Janie offers a strategy for keeping oneself positive all the time:

> I think it's very important to keep your
> mind always positive. I've had to learn it.
> I've found that self-talk helps. I think people
> generally put themselves down a lot, have
> negative thoughts and if you can learn how
> to change the way you think, it can affect
> how your day goes. It can affect everything
> around you. I tried it and it worked.
>
> JANIE, 54

Sharon, 52, puts Janie's idea another way, saying: "We make our own roadblocks, we can knock those roadblocks down."

Stephanie, 49, feels that looking for the bright spots in her day is a survival skill. She explains: "I truly believe that every day there is something positive, one small thing that gives a little bit of spark to your life. If you focus on that ... there can be a lot of unhappy situations that are much easier to deal with." And she shows how finding the bright spots is all in how you look at things: "I look at that box and instead of saying, that's a small box, I say, that's attractive packaging."

Mildred captures the impact a positive outlook has in a particularly memorable way:

> Happiness is like perfume. You sprinkle a
> little on yourself and everyone else smells it.
> And everyone else is enhanced by it.
>
> MILDRED, 64

Strong Sense of Self

It is not easy to come to Health Watch. The women who come sometimes do so despite their own doctor's disapproval. Some of them make long journeys and others get up at incredibly early hours to arrive at their morning appointment in time — some even arrive in Toronto the night before, and stay with friends or family. But come they do. These are women who value themselves, who want to look after themselves. One woman, upon remarking how healthy food might be more expensive, looked me in the eye and said, "I'm worth it." These are women who often literally have to carve out the time needed to do things for themselves. One woman remarked how it was pretty sad, in fact, that she and her friend had to have a doctor's appointment to justify taking a day off from their family responsibilities. These are women who by their presence at Health Watch are saying, "Pay attention to me."

Positive self-esteem is a critical factor in maintaining health. Holistic physician Christiane Northrup has said, "Hope, self-esteem and education are the most important factors in creating health daily." I see that people who feel good about themselves want to take care of themselves. Phyllis, 35, already knows how important a strong sense of self is to health: "You have to be happy about yourself. Just pull up your bootstraps because if you don't, you're just going to be crazy."

Edith, 67 puts the attitude of self-esteem in a nutshell:

I'm very important on this planet, me.

In Conclusion

A healthy diet is one of the keys to health and it is attainable. By eating balanced meals throughout the day, we not only consume both the fuel and nutrients we need, but we free ourselves from uncontrollable evening eating. Balanced eating helps prevent us from gaining large amounts of weight, as long as we include healthy exercise as part of our lifestyle. But our society has become obsessed with weight. It is impossible to avoid the weight issue because we are constantly bombarded by pro-thinness messages from the media, family members, friends and the medical profession. Obesity has been declared the enemy and a war is being waged against it. Many times I have been told by my patients that their doctor told them to lose weight as a solution to their particular health problem. But how good is that advice? Who knows how to successfully take and keep off weight? The generally accepted way of dieting doesn't work. "Why doesn't your doctor advise you to get more exercise?" I ask them. For I am firmly in the camp that promotes health at every weight. Eating healthily and exercising may result in weight loss, but there are no guarantees. I continue to promote healthy habits because studies convincingly show that blood pressure, cholesterol and blood sugar can all be lowered by a healthy lifestyle even if weight is not lost.

Weight is not just a health issue. It is a social issue. We are judged by our size, and the larger we are, the more severe the judgement. As a result, women don't have to be very large before they start feeling concerned about their weight. I have heard the figure mentioned so often that I will jokingly say that the ideal weight for any woman is ten pounds less than she presently weighs. Even when they know that it is impossible to spot reduce, that is, to take weight off in any particular body area, and even when they know that some menopausal weight gain is normal, women pat their tummies at the end of my entreaty to accept their "menopot," and say to me, "I still would like to lose it!"

How can I reconcile this wavering self-esteem my patients show about their weight with the wonderful strong sense of self they show in other areas of their lives? I continually try to link the two in my discussions with my patients. I will continue to try, while acknowledging how small my voice is when compared to the fantastic power of the diet industry.

I acknowledge that many things interfere with people's best intentions to act in healthy ways. I have discussed the major barriers: time restraints, pressures to be thin, and our blind spots around applying knowledge to ourselves. These are major deterrents that no amount of "teaching" can really overcome. People have to make the decision about when to change for themselves. Perhaps self-esteem is the critical factor in change. The women I congratulate for making positive health changes often reply, "I'm trying." And what more can we ask of them? It must be acknowledged that there is no such thing as perfect. There is no perfect diet just as there is no perfect way to live — in fact, I often tell people that I am pretty sure there is no perfect diet because I have been looking for one for years and I have yet to find it. Even if there were a perfect diet, it would be different for each person, because each person is a unique biochemical being.

There are many things we are told to do in order to stay healthy. These include eating well, drinking enough water, exercising, brushing and flossing our teeth, etc. But it's not necessarily possible to fit into one day all the habits that are supposed to maintain health! The women who come to Health Watch make a valiant effort to keep up all these.

But beyond these well known habits that promote health, the women of Health Watch demonstrate an approach and attitude to life that has also been shown to be beneficial. I support the shift away from a medical model of health which limits health practices to diet and exercise and which focuses only on such physical measures as blood pressure, cholesterol and fat intake. Instead, the more holistic approach of the wellness movement recognizes the added health benefit of supportive factors such as purpose in life, social connection and optimism. Wellness encompasses body, mind and spirit. People who have positive attitudes, emotional well-being, healthy human relationships, spirituality and joy live longer and healthier. I believe that the women of Health Watch are included in this group of people. They meditate, pray and reflect. They find ways to relax and to socialize. They have fun, they laugh, they volunteer, they help friends, they dance. They do positive healthy things with a positive healthy attitude and they kindly share their viewpoints with me.

Health Watch has been a two-way street for me. I talk about fuel for our bodies and the women teach me about fuel for their hearts and souls. I believe that life is a process of continual learning and I cannot help but be enriched by interacting with the wise women I see each day. They are strong spirits who truly provide heart and spirit fuel for their lives. I hope that you as the reader have been enriched by the wisdom of the women of Health Watch and that it has touched your spirit as well.

Appendix

Fuel for Healthy Living
As Learned by Miriam from her
Health Watch patients

- Make health a priority.
- Move on — don't dwell. It's okay to stop, reflect, grieve, but eventually life goes on.
- Compare yourself to others to see how fortunate you are.
- Try to think positively.
- Surround yourself with supportive, positive people.
- Keep active.
- Have fun.
- Think about what you have, not about what you don't have.
- Cultivate "healthy fear:" present behaviour affects future health.

I cannot resist making my own contribution to the list:
- Eat your vegetables.

Further Reading

The following is not a comprehensive reading list. My intention, rather, is to highlight some of the books that have either influenced my thinking or made a particular impression on me. I include as well some Web-based resources where more detailed information about nutrition, special diets and exercise is available.

Nutrition

Steven Bratman, *Health Food Junkies,* (Broadway Books, New York, 2000). This book explains how some people get fixated on certain diets, making food more important than it really is.

Adelle Davis, *Let's Eat Right to Keep Fit,* (Harcourt, Brace Jovanovich, Inc., New York, 1970). This book sparked my initial interest in nutrition.

Louise Lambert-Lagace, *Good Nutrition for a Healthy Menopause,* (Stoddart Publishing Co. Limited, Toronto, 1999). One of the best books on nutrition for women.

Roger Williams, *Biochemical Individuality,* (Wiley, New York, 1956). Williams explains in detail the philosophy that we are each unique biochemical beings with different nutritional requirements.

Self-Esteem and Emotional Health

Joan Borysenko, *Guilt is the Teacher, Love is the Lesson,* (Warner Books, Inc., New York, 1990). I recommend this book to patients who are having trouble dealing with guilt feelings.

Carol Johnson, *Self Esteem Comes in All Sizes,* (Doubleday, New York,

1995). This is one of the books that influenced my thinking about the relationship between diets, weight, and self-esteem.

Jon Kabat-Zinn, *Full Catastrophe Living,* (Bantam Doubleday Dell Publishing Group, Inc., New York, 1990). Kabat-Zinn offers in depth information and advice on stress relief, meditation and healing.

Robert Ornstein and David Sobel, *Healthy Pleasures,* (Addison-Wesley Publishing Company, Inc., Don Mills, 1989). This is a wonderful book about healthy pursuits that have nothing to do with diet and exercise.

Rachel Remen, *Kitchen Table Wisdom,* (The Berkeley Publishing Group, New York, 1996). My very favourite book — it also has nothing to do with diet or exercise, but is all about nourishing the self.

Internet Resources

- For information about the non-dieting approach to life, check out the Healthy Weight Journal Web site, www.healthyweightnetwork.com, and www.hugs.com.

- To get a copy of Canada's Food Guide to Healthy Eating go to www.hc-sc.gc.ca/hppb/nutrition/pbe/foodguide/index.html.

- To get a copy of Canada's Physical Activity Guide to Healthy Active Living go to www.hc-sc.gc.ca/english/lifestyles/physical_activity.html.

- For information on healthy eating and Web resources on a variety of diet and nutrition topics, visit www.dialadietitian.org.

- To find a dietitian near you and for nutrition information, contact the Dietitians of Canada at www.dietitians.ca.